DO IT
OR
AGE QUICKLY

60-second practices to live better, stronger, and longer

JB Berns

Published by Urban Productions, Inc.

Cover design by Pauline Neuwirth.
Interior design and illustrations by Lisa Weistroffer.

Disclaimer: While every effort has been taken to ensure the accuracy and effectiveness of the information in this book, Urban Productions, Inc., makes no guarantee, express or implied, as to the procedures contained herein. Neither the author nor publisher will be liable for direct, indirect, incidental, or consequential damages in connection with or arising from the furnishing, performance, or use of this book.

Reference in this book to a trademark, proprietary product, or company name is intended for explicit description only and does not imply approval or recommendation to the exclusion of others that may be suitable.

This book is not meant to replace the professional advice and expertise of your physician, or to encourage patients to evaluate risks and benefits of using medications, supplements, products, nutritional advice, exercises, and treatments without considering their healthcare provider.

ISBN 978-0-578-05833-7

Printed and bound in the United States of America.

SPECIAL THANKS

The author gratefully wishes to give special thanks to the following people:

Irvin Berns
Linda Berns
Stephen T. Chang, M.D.
Jonathan Flaum
Kow Loon Ong

ACKNOWLEDGEMENTS

Beth Berns
Penni Berns
John Campbell
Rich Celaya
Chris Chin
Christopher Esposito
Jim Hornbeck
Ron Jason
Kenny Karlowitz
Robin Kopit
Stanley Kopit
Gary Lutz
Dan Millman
Daniel Reid
Randolph San Millan
Scott Silberman
Lanny Taylor
Paul Williams

TABLE OF CONTENTS

ABOUT THE AUTHOR

JB Berns has a long background in the martial arts, yoga, personal and wellness training, and developing exercise systems. He was named by *Fitness Magazine* in 1999 as one of the top 10 personal trainers in the nation. While recovering from a knee injury, he used his 20-plus years of martial arts experience to develop the low-impact Urban Rebounder exercise system, selling millions and having *Consumer Reports* call it one of the top 100 products in 2008. The Urban Rebounder is now in over 5,000 gyms worldwide and 18 different countries. JB has also created many DVDs for exercise and wellness, which are available worldwide in nine different languages, including *The Perfect Martial Arts Workout*, *Rehab Your Body at Home*, *The Isometric Total Body Workout*, *Deante Modern Dance Workouts*, and *Kids Bound* (Urban Rebounding for children). In addition, he designed the Jackie Chan Cable-Flex System for resistance and aerobic exercise at home. JB is the author of *Urban Rebounder: An Exercise for the New Millennium* and has appeared on the *Today Show*, CNN, CBS, NBC, *The View*, and *The Doctors*.

INTRODUCTION

In my 20-plus years of martial and yogic training, I learned about practices and products from my many instructors that I was urged to put into place in my daily routine. I listened. I incorporated them into my life because they were simple techniques that took no time at all, made me feel great, and, I was told, would keep me healthy and slow down the aging process. Those instructors are now in their 70s, 80s, and 90s and literally look half their age and are in amazing shape. I wrote this book at the insistence of my clients and friends to now bring those techniques to you.

This book contains a system of 21 simple anti-aging techniques that most people have not heard of before. I will tell you about a hair preservation routine for men, natural toothpaste that whitens teeth and doesn't strip away your enamel, herbal tea that energizes and bolsters your immune system, facial creams that are better than anything on the market that heal and preserve your skin, stress and fear-reducing methods, a consumption routine that streamlines digestion and brings about effortless weight loss, and stretches and exercises that take only 60 seconds each. In fact, the beauty of this book, as you can probably tell from the title, is that each of my 21 recommendations takes only 60 seconds!

My system is easy, and fun, and anyone can do it. I cannot emphasize enough how much it has changed and benefited my life. It has given me a positive approach to life and helps me start my day with a smile, every day. I have defied the genetics of my family who have male pattern baldness, I am in top physical condition with little effort, and despite a busy, demanding life in New York City, my stress level is negligible—to name just a few effects.

Buying this book is a very small investment in what it can do for your life. Please give it a try—why not? The products I advocate are natural, available, and affordable. My advice for harnessing the power of your mind can benefit your outlook as well as your health. The stretches and exercises can be done by most anyone, including someone who has never exercised or has physical limitations. Some of my advice you can actually do in your sleep.

Influences

Many influences shaped this book—many philosophies and many what you might call philosophers. They all contributed a unique vision and inspiration, yet they are all unified in many core aspects.

As a martial artist for more than half of my life, this discipline has affected not only my view of physical activity but of mental involvement as well. It trained me to engage my mind while using my body, thus exercising both realms at once. It also introduced me to free-form movement as a physical activity, as opposed to monotonous exercises that chain you to specific movements. Many of the practices in this book are in a similar vein. They are efficient exercises that take little time and yet utilize the power of the mind. Body, mind, and spirit are in balance, which is our ultimate goal.

Because I am interested in the latter, it was natural that I would embrace Taoism, where balance, harmony, and effortlessness of natural processes provide a model for human action.

Taoism encompasses principles of the body, diet, breathing, physical exercises, use of herbs, and meditation, practices that have held up for the Chinese for thousands of years and bring one closer to the natural order of things. The classic text of Taoism, the *Tao Te Ching*, was, according to tradition, written in the sixth century BC and lays the foundation of Taoism. This has greatly influenced my life philosophy. You will see this throughout the text when I discuss the importance of achieving balance in life, as it deeply affects the quality of your life, whether you are able to balance time, energy, work, family, friends, and relaxation. There is a focus on maximizing the power of your energy flow and ensuring that it is functioning properly to heal and protect your health. And finally I emphasize the practice of emptying your mind as Taoists do, so you can focus on the practices at hand.

This brings me to meditation and breathing exercises, which have also influenced me and are prevalent in this book. I believe that meditation (including visualization) and focusing on your breathing are a way to achieve harmony and balance in your life, as well as a means to achieving your life goals. It seems like such a simple thing, but it is fundamental to everything else. (Please read Chapter 2, Ten Deep Breaths, for more information and guidance.)

I also owe much credit to the remarkable instructors and mentors in my life. Mr. Kow Loon Ong (Kayo) is a master teacher in the fine art of Okinawan Goju kara-te and has been a teacher, role model, and personal friend of mine since 1987. He is a martial artist in the purist sense, only concerned about the craft and the art of it, not commercializing or profiting from his teaching but taking it to underprivileged children and so on. This system of kara-te mimics the white crane, and when you watch this man perform it, he is so accomplished, he *is* a white crane. He takes the art from the dojo (training hall) to the outside and into your everyday life. I owe him very much for this gift.

Dr. Stephen T. Chang is another instructor who has had a profound influence in my life and ways of thinking. He is a practicing master Taoist, herbalist, and M.D., and the author of several powerful books that have changed my life. (See the epilogue for more information on this.) After many years of reading his work, attending his workshops, and conversing with him as I have gotten to know him personally, it is my great honor to relay the essence of his most important teachings to you. Dr. Chang's guidance and teachings can change anyone's life for the better.

I am also indebted to the master yoga instructor who brought Ashtanga yoga to the Western world, Sri K. Pattabhi Jois. He was a wise and humble man who spryly taught yoga into his 90s until his recent death. Jois taught an ancient system that combined movement with focused breathing in order to build unity with the mind, body, and spirit. He also taught that his exercises were for everyone, even those with busy lives, work, and family. I embrace all of these concepts in this book as well. As he was based in India, I was fortunate enough to be taught by Jois' student, John Campbell.

The following people I will discuss more quickly, but they have had no less positive impact upon my life than the previous three. Dan Millman is the author of many wonderful books including *The Way of the Peaceful Warrior*. His workshop in 1987 opened my heart and soul. Paul Williams, author of *Das Energi*, has written a timeless tome that every man and woman should read before turning 30. His book was an inspiration in many ways and the basis for Chapter 20, The Five Rules to Conquer Fear. And finally, Daniel Reid is a

Taoist herbalist and the author of the amazing book *The Tao of Health, Sex and Longevity*. This book has essentially been a road map for me to live my life better, stronger, and longer.

In summary, my beliefs and influences are in free-form exercise that engage both the mind and the body, the use of deep breathing and emptying the mind of everything but the present, a disciplined system that doesn't overwhelm you but can become a fluid and vital part of your life, and action-oriented exercises designed to bring balance to all areas of your life, be it physical or mental, in work and at home.

The System

In years past I have done my best to pass on the knowledge from all of my extraordinary teachers to my clients, friends, and family. They pleaded with me to write it all down in a handy reference guide, so that is what I have attempted to do here. I have gathered together all of my most valuable teachings over the years, practices that will transform your days and slow down the aging process. I systemized it and put it into an easy-to-follow daily formula.

Performing all of the practices in the book every day would be ideal, but doing some or only a few each day would also be adequate. I don't believe in marathon workouts or straining yourself to perform these exercises—that defeats the purpose. It can't be extreme if it's going to fit into your life. Your physical activity should be balanced, as should your mind. It's the process we're concerned with, about the action of doing. The chapters in this book are only a springboard. What will really change your life is doing it: as the yoga guru Jois used to say, "It's 1% theory, and 99% practice." He also preached action and patience: "Practice and all is coming." And the sign of a *Peaceful Warrior*, as author Dan Millman would say, "Is one who acts and does not react."

Just do it. Put it into practice and try these time-tested (for centuries!) practices. The exercises are simple, the products are natural and non-toxic, and years may be added to your life. Just do it.

The Power of 21

For most people there is a lot of new information between the covers of this book. How are you going to remember what to do every day? Even though each recommendation has been distilled down to its essence in the 60-second box that begins each chapter, there are still 21 steps to remember as you go about your day. The Power of 21 is setting up the system for following the 21 60-second anti-aging practices.

What I recommend is to review the Table of Contents each day. Try to incorporate as many practices into your daily routine as you can. Some may take longer than 60 seconds in the beginning; it may take a little while until you're familiar and comfortable with everything. Pick your favorite practices and build from there. Now, the key is, do this for 21 days. There is something magical and transforming about doing something for 21 days. Whatever you keep doing for that period will form a habit. A switch goes off, and what you once had to remind yourself to do becomes reflexive and a part of your conscious and subconscious routine. (Just be careful what you repeat, because negative activities can become habits, too!)

The power of 21 has significant value to me because of my experience doing things 21 times in a row. I sincerely believe that if an individual repeats something or does something 21 days in a row (and I hope that activity is positive for one's spirit) the process will become part of his or her "basic self." What I mean by "basic self" is that the movement or exercise will become a normal part of your everyday activities without adding any stress to your life. To further define what I mean, you'll look forward to doing the 21 practices in this book—hopefully not only 21 days in a row, but throughout your life.

The first time I experienced the power of the number 21 was over 20 years ago when one of my teachers, Dan Millman (*Way of the Peaceful Warrior*), stated to me in one of his workshops, "JB, don't ask so many questions, just do the movement or the activity with the correct spirit, with the body and mind connected as a union 21 times, and all your questions will be answered." (1% theory, 99% practice!) And how right Mr. Dan Millman was.

Remember that you do not have to do all 21 practices 21 days in a row. You can choose which ones are of higher priority or those which apply specifically to your life, although I do urge you to have trust in me and try all of them for 21 days in a row. And do keep in mind that the 21 pattern of repetition can also apply to negative activities to weaken one's spirit; for example, if you smoked cigarettes or lost your temper 21 days in a row, the power of 21, the repetition of 21 would still apply. I once heard from a past instructor that the power of 21 and its repetition had something to do with astrology and the alignment of the earth's axis, but sincerely, my friends, I'm not concerned with that. I feel if you do a task for 21 days in a row (hopefully the 21 practices in this book), it is enough of a repetition to become internalized in your being and spirit.

In Closing

I have done all of the research for you, the reader. My instructors and theirs have time-tested each practice and chapter.

Just go do it and make it a part of your Basic Self, a part of your Being. Just go do it and practice the practices, and all is coming. Do you have 60 seconds to live a new life—one that will be better, stronger, and longer?

1

CORRECT POSTURE: ASLEEP AND AWAKE

For 60 Seconds:
Go to sleep in the proper position; keep your back straight while awake.

People tend to sacrifice much of their everyday energy and restorative possibilities of sleep by applying unhealthy forms of posture. In this chapter I will instruct you on proper posture positions while you are both asleep and awake in order to maximize your natural energy.

Asleep

Given that the average person spends approximately a third of his or her life sleeping, it should come as no surprise that the position you sleep in can have a significant impact on your overall health.

It's best to lie on your back while you sleep, as this position does not put any undue pressure on your internal organs, and your heart in particular is unencumbered. Sleeping on your back also allows your airways to be free and clear for full oxygen exchange, and it helps preserve your facial skin, as it is not creased during the night. If you switch to this position, it may take some time to feel comfortable—but don't give up, because better rest and bodily functioning will be the end result.

Sleeping on your right side is the next best position, as it has been associated with lowering sympathetic nervous activity, which is what controls heart rate and blood pressure. When

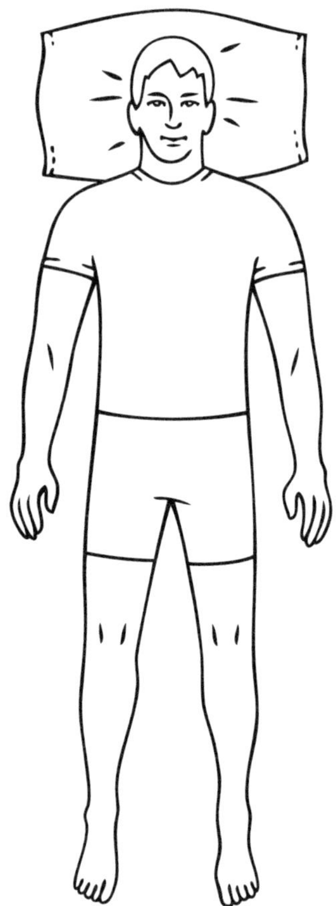

FIGURE 1. The ideal sleeping position: sleeping on your back.

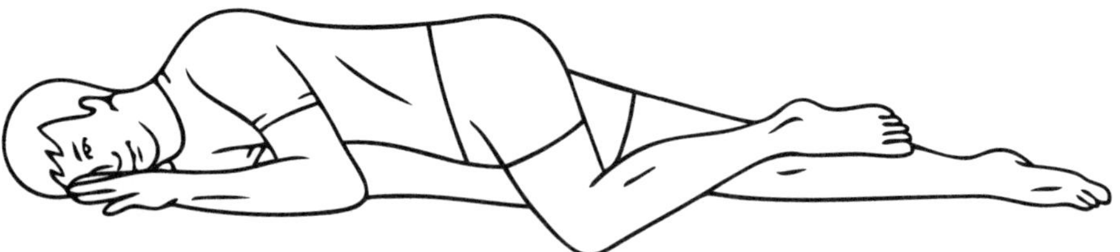

FIGURE 2. Correct sleeping position when sleeping on the right side.

the right side is down, the heart is in a more superior position, which may make it easier for it to pump blood out.

Because the heart is positioned more to the left side in most people, lying on your left side may compress the heart somewhat (as compared to lying on your right side), thus impeding its function.

Avoid sleeping on your stomach. This position increases pressure on your lungs, diaphragm, heart, and internal organs, resulting in diminished function and shallower breathing. Sleeping this way with a pillow overarches the natural curve of the back and can create back pain as well as restless sleep. Furthermore, because this sleeping posture forces you to twist your head to the side, neck pain can result.

I can attest to the transformation that can take place from sleeping with correct posture. For many years my sleep was disturbed from my heart beating hard in the middle of the night, and I would wake up in the morning with a heaviness in my chest. I didn't know what it was from. I went to several cardiologists in pursuit of the answer—I had EKGs, stress tests, and so on, and they said everything was fine. They didn't know how to help me. Then I went to a seminar where I heard Dr. Stephen T. Chang talk about sleep postures and patterns. Dr. Chang is an M.D. and also a practitioner of ancient Chinese medicine. He melds the wisdom and experience of thousands of years of Taoist health practices with a modern understanding of how physiology and energy flow function. It turned out the answer was as simple as going to sleep in a different position: don't sleep on your left side because of pressure on your heart, don't sleep on your stomach because of pressure on your internal organs, sleep on your right side or your back, and that's it. No treatments or prescription drugs. Immediately after trying it, the heaviness I had experienced in the morning, as well as the insomnia from my heart beating harder, had disappeared. I realize it can be difficult to change because you're used to the sleeping habits you've had for umpteen years, but trust me, the benefits are significant. You owe it to yourself to get a wonderful, restful good night's sleep.

Awake

Sitting Position

You can improve your health and energy just by sitting correctly. The best way to sit is on the floor with one or (preferably) both hips pivoted out. See the following figures for the correct sitting position with both hips open (cross-legged) and with one (one leg extended out). These amazing postures will open up your hips and increase circulation. In the Far East and Middle East very few people have hip problems or hip replacements. This is because most of the time the people in these cultures are sitting on the floor and not in a Western chair that slows circulation to the middle of the body and

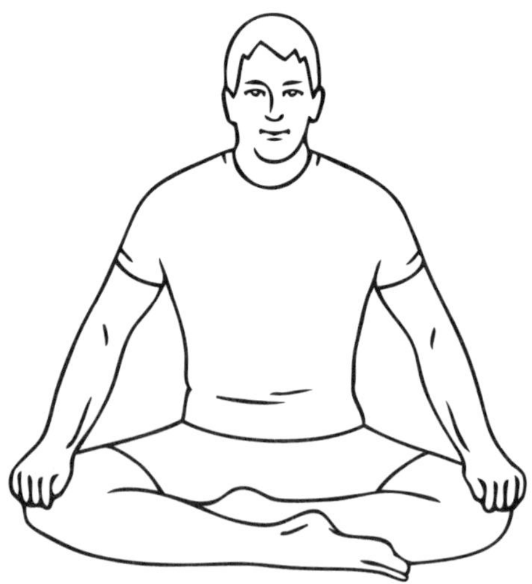

FIGURE 3. Correct sitting posture in the cross-legged position.

hip area. The Western chair essentially pinches your hips and does not allow you to open them as you can do on the floor. Because of this, I strongly suggest you sit on the floor in the positions I describe whenever possible. Personally, when I have no choice but to sit in a Western chair, I usually have one hip out, resting one foot up on my chair to open up the circulation. The more you do this, the better the health of your hips and knees, and the lesser the chance you will suffer problems with them later on.

While by far the best position is to sit on the floor, if you need to sit in a chair, your back should be erect, thighs parallel to the floor, and feet flat on the floor. Better yet, sit as I do, shown in the following figure, opening up at least one of your legs.

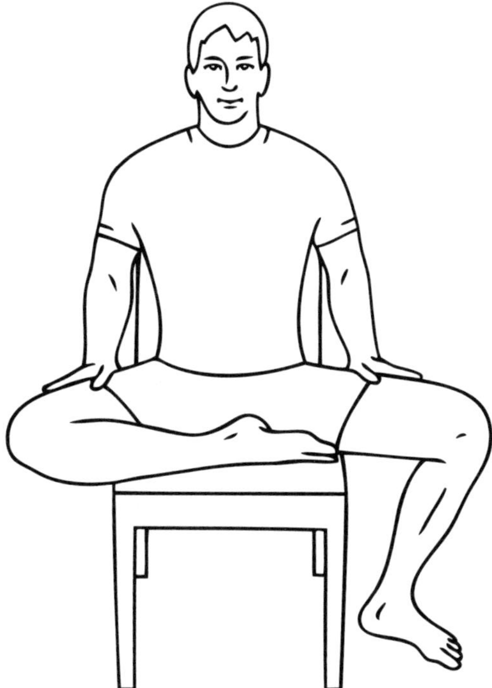

FIGURE 4. Recommended posture while sitting down on a chair or similar object.

You can also increase energy in your body by sitting on the floor. By bending at least one leg in, you can press your heel into your prostate gland or clitoris to protect and energize the sexual organs. The sexual organs are the most fundamental glands of the body, so they require special attention. Energizing them creates more energy for your body as a whole. You can achieve a similar effect by either sitting in the position shown below, with one heel pressing while the other is extended, or with a hard object such as a ball pressing against you. Any of these positions are recommended whenever possible when you are sitting, including during Internal Exercises, meditation, deep breathing, work, reading, and so on.

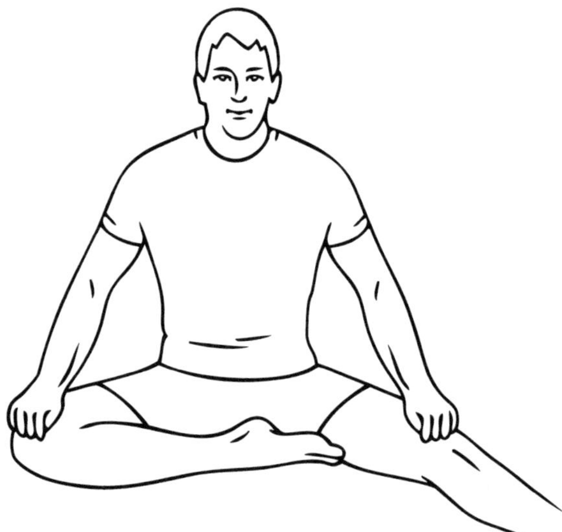

FIGURE 5. Sitting position with one heel pressing in, one leg extended.

Standing Position

The best standing position is demonstrated in the following figure. Stand with feet parallel to each other, shoulder-width apart. Keep your back straight and stand evenly on your two feet. This position will help keep your mind alert and give your body a feeling of lightness.

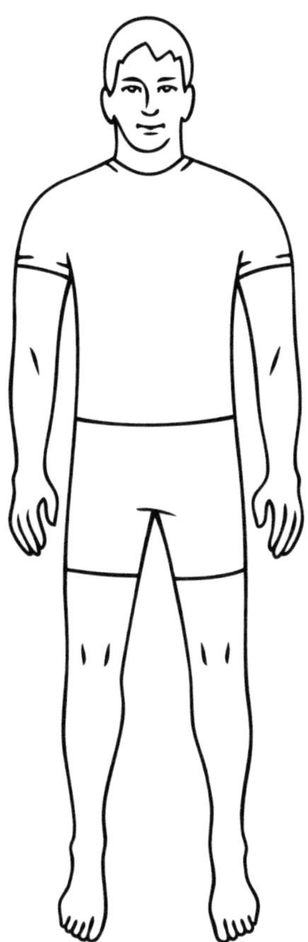

FIGURE 6. Correct standing position.

Note: *If you have medical concerns such as neck or back pain, sleep apnea, or gastroesophageal reflux, consult your physician for the best sleep position for you.*

For more information on posture, go to:
www.DOITORAGEQUICKLY.com
www.JBBERNS.com

2

TEN DEEP BREATHS

For 60 Seconds:
Take 10 long, deep breaths when you wake up in the morning.

Deep breathing has long been considered essential for maintaining chi, the life-force energy of Eastern cultural traditions. Only more recently, however, have Americans begun to embrace the wisdom of taking a deep breath. I am a big proponent of taking the time and concentration to breathe deeply for a period of time every day. In fact, it is probably the most important advice I have for you, and one of the most fundamental things you should be doing every day. The benefits are copious, both helping the body and the mind.

Stress is related to breathing, and breathing is related to stress. If you are stressed, you tend to breathe faster, shallower breaths. This deprives your body of oxygen saturation, which could contribute to many illnesses and conditions, such as high blood pressure and congestive heart failure. I feel that the only difference between fear and excitement is breathing. When you're fearful, your breathing is very shallow. When you're excited, your breathing is very quick and unpredictable. Both of these states contribute to increased stress upon your body. However, practicing slow, deep breathing exercises can by itself help reduce stress. So which is easier to change, the situations in your life that create stress, or focusing on how you breathe, which you have to do anyway? The answer is obvious.

Let me give you some practical examples of when the power of the breath can be applied. Maybe you're driving in your car and you're really frustrated from a traffic jam, or from someone cutting you off without a signal or wave. Or you're having an argument with someone. Or you're waiting in line. Or you're slogging through an automated menu on the telephone, or dealing with any number of modern annoyances and inconveniences. If you try the ten-deep-breaths technique I describe for you below, I assure you, you will be less agitated—rather, the 10 deep breaths will have an overall calming effect to your being. So I suggest anytime you get frustrated at all, try taking 10 deep breaths for 60 seconds. It just might change your outlook and your behavior in these stressful situations.

With practice, the breath work you do will quiet down your nervous system. This will not only blunt anxiety but also lower your blood pressure, slow your heart rate, improve your circulation and digestion, and help protect your body from the damaging effects of stress. In terms of the benefits from the breathing technique itself, fully oxygenating your body is beneficial for all systems throughout your body. Breathing oxygenates every cell of your body, from your brain to your vital organs. Without sufficient oxygen, your body becomes more susceptible to health problems. For example, in a study published in *The Lancet*, cardiac patients who took faster, shallower breaths per minute were more likely to have low levels of blood oxygen. This gave them a poorer prognosis for their condition. It might also impair skeletal muscle and metabolic function and lead to muscle atrophy and exercise intolerance. The patients who learned a slow breathing technique improved their oxygen saturation, exercise tolerance, and prognosis.

Deep breathing may also benefit the lymphatic system because it depends on the muscular movement of breathing to move lymph throughout your body. The lymphatic system works to remove extra fluid from tissues and cells and transports away the waste products of blood, absorbs and transports fats to the circulatory system, and filters harmful microorganisms and abnormal cells from your body. The fluid is then transported back into the bloodstream via lymph vessels.

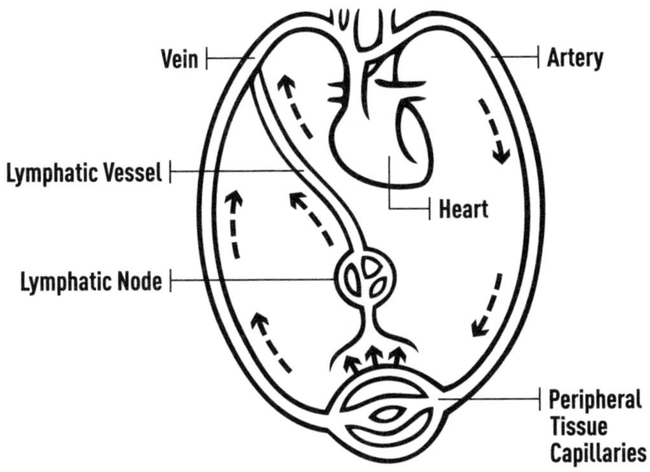

FIGURE 7. The lymphatic system works in conjunction with the circulatory system to transport waste and toxins from your body.

The consequence of a sluggish lymphatic system is that you cannot filter out waste products as effectively and your immune system will not function at capacity. If you aren't breathing deeply or moving regularly, chances are your lymph fluid is not flowing as well as it could be either.

The great news is that you can improve your lymph system cleansing by learning to practice deep breathing. The expansion and contraction of the diaphragm actually stimulate your lymphatic system and massages your internal organs, maximizing the removal of toxins, foreign invaders, and even cancer cells, while promoting an optimal exchange of oxygen.

Here is a summary of some of the amazing, therapeutic benefits of deep breathing (for more information, see *The Tao of Health, Sex, & Longevity* by Daniel P. Reid):

- **Respiration:** The diaphragm is the muscle that lines the bottom of the lungs and upon contraction and release is responsible for the inhalation and exhalation of the lungs. Deep breathing strengthens, stretches, and tones the diaphragm. This in turn increases inhalation capacity and oxygen intake, improves breath control, and deepens abdominal massage. The effect deep breathing has on increasing the volume of oxygen intake and decreasing the number of breaths can last for several hours after performing the exercises.
- **Circulation:** Extended periods of deep breathing (e.g., 20–30 minutes) can have tremendous benefits for the heart and circulatory system. Your pulse is slowed, saving heartbeats, and the amount of red blood cells (responsible for delivering oxygen to your body) dramatically increases.
- **Digestion:** Digestion, metabolism, and excretion are greatly improved due to the excitation of the pneumogastric nerve that occurs during deep breathing. The automatic massage the diaphragm performs upon the stomach and liver improves digestion and promotes peristalsis.
- **Hormonal secretions:** As I have said, the reproductive organs are an important foundation of our body's overall health.

Hence, the fact that deep breathing stimulates vital hormonal secretions throughout the endocrine system is quite significant. The excitation of the pneumogastric nerve stimulates the endocrine system, which provides direct massage to glands in the abdomen and sacrum. Essentially, deep breathing indirectly helps balance all vital functions, including strengthening the reproductive organs and bolstering sexual potency and fertility.

- **Sleep:** Deep breathing can improve your sleep, and indirectly improve your waking hours as well. It permits deep, uninterrupted sleep and maximizes sleep so you can feel completely rested with fewer hours of sleep.
- **Stress reduction:** As I have touched on in some detail above, deep breathing calms stressful emotions and brings them under conscious control. Practicing a few deep breaths at the moment of great stress can bring the body back into equilibrium, and the mind will follow as well.
- **Mental acuity:** Mental faculties such as awareness, thought, and memory are greatly enhanced by deep breathing. It can improve your state of mind at any given moment.

The technique is as simple as taking 10 long, deep breaths. It can be done lying down, standing, or in a seated position. While taking the 10 deep breaths, you may try putting your right or left pointer finger inside your belly button (either on bare skin or over your shirt) if you like; this will connect all energies from the hand to the navel and allow you to get in touch with your body as well as listen to your pulse.

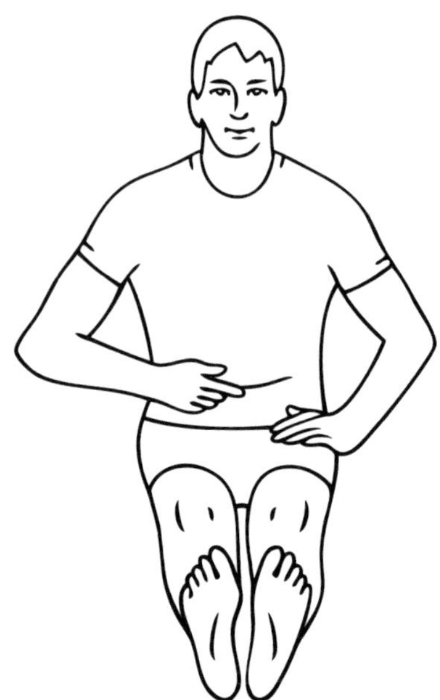

FIGURE 8. One position for deep breathing exercises.

You can also perform the breathing exercises cross-legged with your arms resting at your hips, or leaning against a wall or headboard, as shown in the following figures.

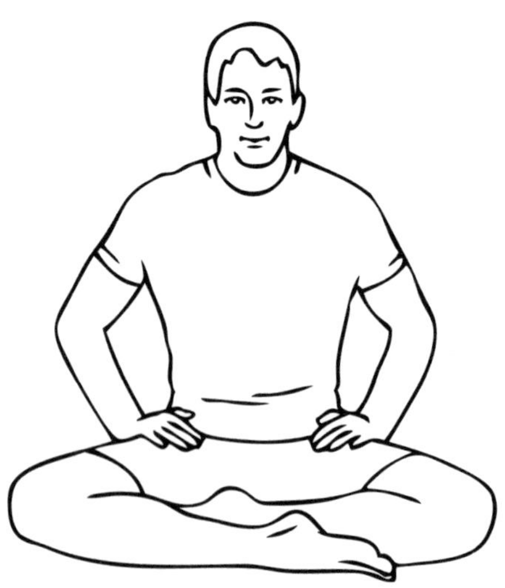

FIGURE 9. Another position for deep breathing exercises.

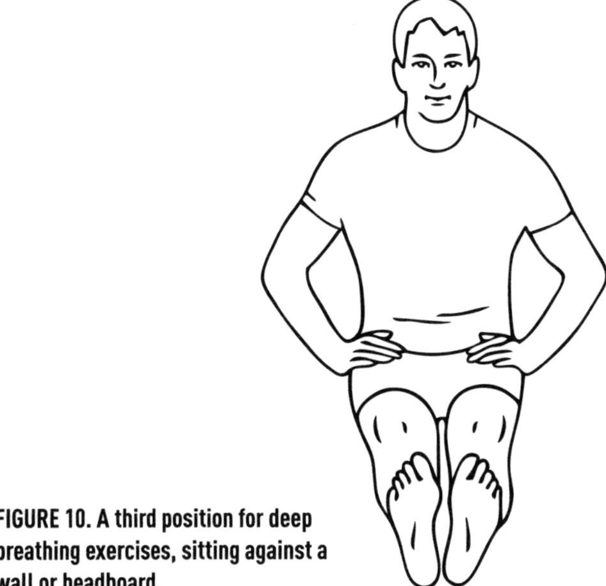

FIGURE 10. A third position for deep breathing exercises, sitting against a wall or headboard.

Focus on your posture while you take your 10 deep breaths. I recommend the following four-step approach:

1. First, take a deep breath in through your nose while gently resting your tongue on the roof of your mouth.
2. Squeeze your perineum/anal muscles, while simultaneously pushing your tongue against the roof of your mouth—this way the tongue acts as your body's natural electrical ground for added balance and concentration.
3. Hold your breath for the same number of seconds it took you to inhale.
4. Exhale out through your nose (again, for the same number of seconds you inhaled and held your breath). At the same time, release the perineum lock, and stop pushing your tongue against the roof of your mouth. Your tongue should

remain resting gently on the top of your mouth as you get ready for your next inhale.

You may not be able to execute 10 particularly long breaths right away. To build up, first try to count to one, then two, as many as you can do. Keep the motion fluid. Increase the number each week, and over time your lung capacity will increase to the point that the exercise is effortless.

I recommend doing this when you awake in the morning. That way your day is started on a positive, relaxed note, thus helping the rest of your day to follow in this manner. In addition, you are less likely to forget to do it if you incorporate it into your morning routine. I also recommend doing the exercise before each meal during the day and at night before bed.

Breath work is a natural segue to meditation, because the simplest meditation technique is concentration on the breath. In Taoism, methods of meditation and breathing are utilized to augment the energy in one's body, to keep a constant flow of energy in the body for ultimate health and longevity, and as a tool for observing inner states of weakness, vulnerability, and disease.

The association of meditation with Eastern religion is an obstacle for some Americans, but many nonreligious forms exist. In essence, meditation is nothing other than focused awareness. It's not absolutely necessary, but I do recommend that you incorporate meditation into your deep breathing routine at least now and then if you can—give it a try.

Every day when I perform yoga postures or martial arts movements, I always concentrate on my breath. This focuses my mind on my breath as well as on what I am doing. If I don't do this, my mind begins to wander. When I was a young kid in the martial arts, I could never do this and never understood what the union of the body and mind was. Now I understand so clearly that it is connecting your breath to the physical movement of your body, or the lack thereof when there is no movement at all and you are in a state of true stillness. Some call this meditation. But you must remember, you don't have to be still to meditate. You can be moving or walking and still be meditating, as long as you are focused and aware and in tune with your breath.

The focus on your breath and on your actions go hand in hand. I try to perform difficult postures and exercises such as a handstand derived from a full split. If I do not use the power of my mind to visualize my feet together in a handstand, coupled with utter awareness of my breath, the probability of me not performing this very difficult maneuver is increased. Ten deep breaths, my friends, in whatever posture, seated or standing, when you awake. And I hope throughout the day. The most important thing in my life is the power of my breath.

Throughout the day, stop what you're doing for 60 seconds, focus, and take ten long, deep breaths—you will feel the change in your life. Wouldn't it be great if we all breathed as deeply during the day as when we slept?

For more information on deep breathing, go to:
www.DOITORAGEQUICKLY.com
www.JBBERNS.com

3

INTERNAL EXERCISES

For 60 Seconds:
Perform your internal exercises
(they may seem external to you, but they're not).

I believe this chapter on exercising one's internal organs contains some of the most important advice in my book. It may be a foreign concept to many people, but I truly believe that these exercises can invigorate you on a daily basis, help heal ailing organs, and protect you from disease for long-term health and longevity. My mentor and teacher of many years, Dr. Stephen Chang, brought these amazing life-transforming exercises to me, and I implore you to try them and incorporate them into your daily routine.

The internal exercises were created by ancient Taoists over time through careful study and application of the physical laws of nature, exhaustively observing the animal kingdom, and analyzing the natural principles of healing. They believed that the physical laws they observed in nature held true for the human body also—and that they could use the same theories and systems to coax diseased parts of a body back to their natural state of being. Thus, the internal exercises were born. By performing them daily, you should be able to live your life free of disease and pain, which is the natural state for your body to be in. In addition, they bring about a wonderful sense of well-being that springs from the heart of each individual, something I can definitely attest to happening.

The main emphasis of the internal exercises is on strengthening your body and your mind. Preventive medicine, if you will. The goal is to tone all of the internal systems, including the emotional and the spiritual. The exercises also help us cope with stresses—environmental, social, and internal. We should achieve a state of harmony with our minds at peace and our bodies healthy. Everything is connected, one organ to the other, and our minds to our bodies. Energy is the foundation of it all, and it flows through our body in a continuum.

The Taoist internal exercises Dr. Chang has detailed in his book, *The Complete System of Self-Healing: Internal Exercises*, have been a pure gift from him to me. I could never thank him enough for what they have done for my life and my health. When I awake every morning, some of the first things I do are the internal exercises described in this chapter. My entire body feels warm, refreshed, and energized after completing them. It's almost as if I've had a full-body massage, except that it is so much better than coming from a therapist, because I am using my own body's healing power.

While the internal exercises are so simple they can be carried out anytime, anywhere, there is a rare day here and there that I skip them. But when I am too busy and do not slow down and perform the exercises, the result is a very sluggish day and my energy is very low. I strongly encourage you to do them every day! It's easy, and they are so much fun to do!

Internal Exercises

You can do these exercises anywhere because all you need for them are your hands. Although you can do them at any time of day, and I often feel like doing that myself, I do recommend that you do them in the morning. They are best done completely disrobed (or at least with your shirt off), so it's probably easier to do them before you dress for the day.

Before starting the internal exercises, I recommend that you rub your hands together firmly to create friction, and then immediately apply your hand to the body part you intend to work. Start with the top of your body—your head—and work down, although, as you will see, the order is not strictly head to toe. In all of these exercises it is essential to focus on what you are doing and not let your mind wander. Always breathe slowly, and try to experience the energy flow.

Below is my list of internal exercises that you should perform every day (instructions and diagrams to follow).

1. Head
2. Eyes
3. Nose
4. Ears
5. Mouth
6. Neck and Thyroid
7. Lungs
8. Heart
9. Stomach
10. Liver
11. Kidneys
12. Arms
13. Legs
14. Head Hanging
15. Internal Organ Relaxation

1. Head

Kneading pressure applied by massage warms the skin and opens up blood vessels to increase flow and boost circulation. Increased circulation on the scalp means that the cells of the hair follicle will receive more of the nutrients necessary for optimal hair growth function and keeps the hair from falling out. To properly do this exercise, place your fingers on top of your head as shown in the following drawing, and press your fingers down. Rub your skin back and forth without lifting your hands from your head, pressing with moderate to firm pressure, increasing the intensity as the weeks progress. Be careful not to scratch yourself while doing it.

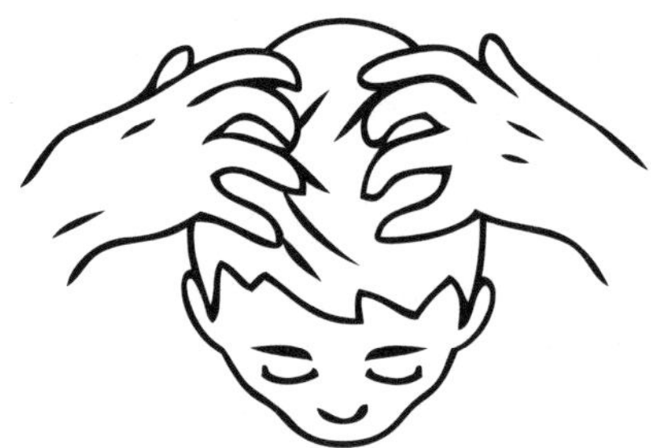

FIGURE 11. Scalp massage.

Because this exercise opens up blood vessels that flow to the scalp, and starts the circulation moving there, you will feel a tingling on your scalp.

Next, press your thumbs onto the back of your neck as indicated (see following figure). Press in firmly and rub at the same time. This exercise is designed to remove tension and fatigue from the upper back and neck, so it may help eliminate or prevent tension headaches.

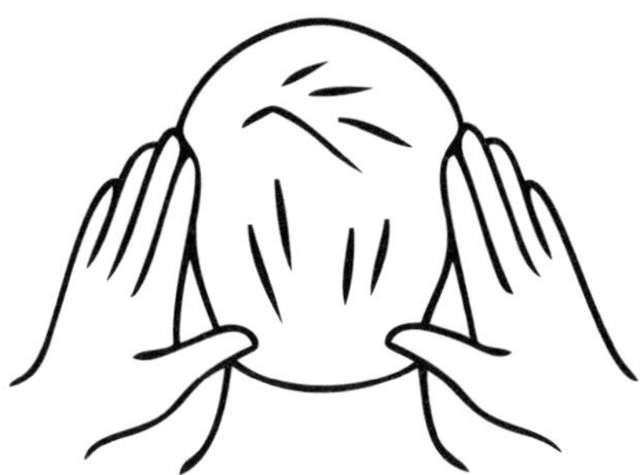

FIGURE 12. Neck massage for tension and fatigue.

2. Eyes

Massaging your eyes will benefit vision, as well as cosmetic appearance, as it reduces bags or puffiness under your eyes. Dark circles under your eyes are a sign of poor circulation, which can also be helped by these exercises.

The following figure identifies the five acupressure points of the eye.

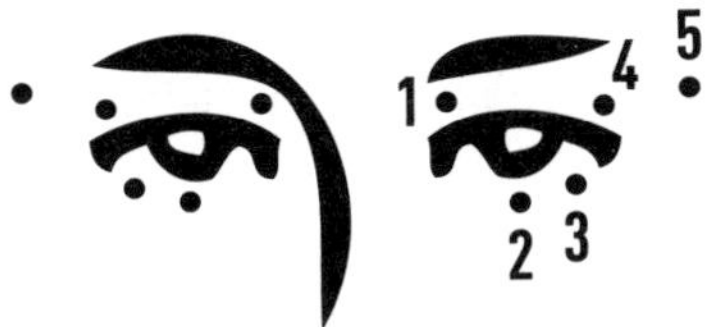

FIGURE 13. The five acupressure points of the eye.

For the first exercise, see point 1 above. Place your thumbs here, on the rims of the eye sockets at the upper inside corner of the eyes (see the following figure). There is a slight depression in the bone at the correct spot. Press in deeply and massage the spots for a count of 10, then release. Repeat for a total of three times. Any pain indicates blockage (poor blood flow); massage lightly whenever you feel pain.

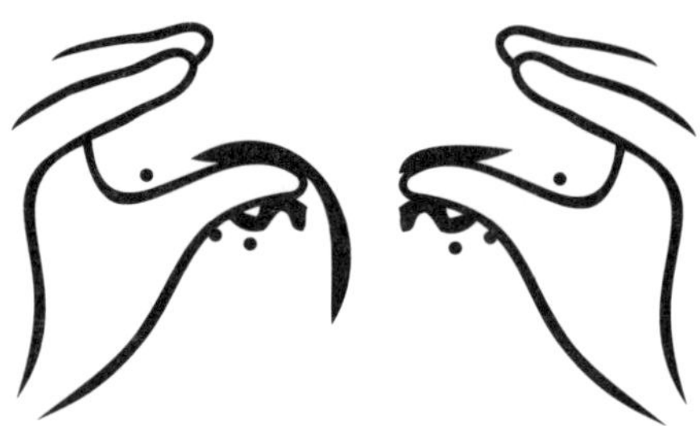

FIGURE 14.
Massaging acupressure point 1.

For the second exercise, place your index fingers at point 2—in the small depressions at the middle of the lower eye sockets (see following figure). Press in deeply on the rims of the eye sockets (not the cheekbones) for a count of 10, release. Repeat for a total of three times.

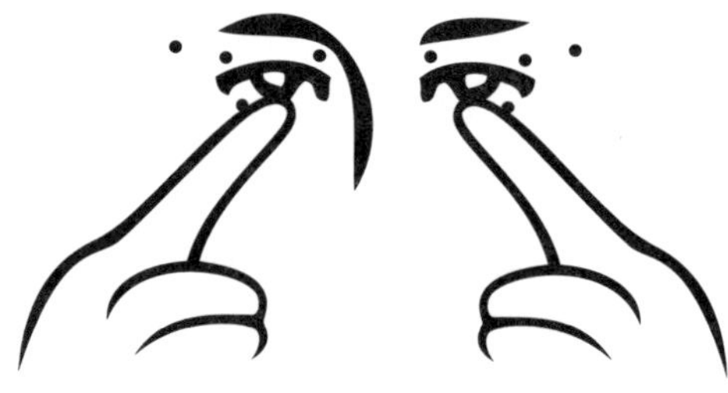

FIGURE 15.
Massaging acupressure point 2.

For the third exercise, place your index fingers at point 3, on the lower eye socket one-quarter of the way in from the outside corners of your eyes (see following figure). Press and massage for a count of 10 and release. Repeat for a total of three times.

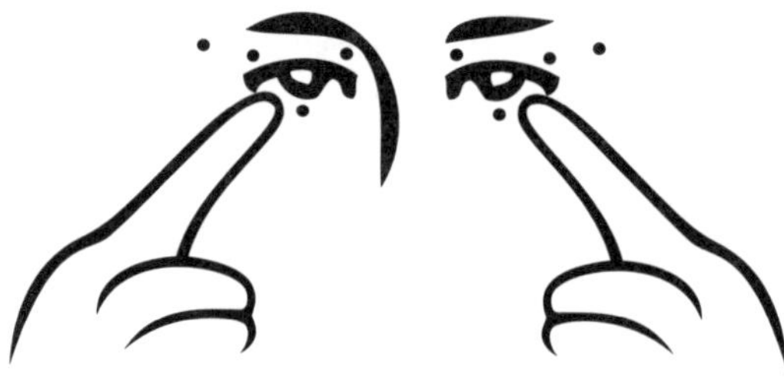

FIGURE 16.
Massaging acupressure point 3.

For the next exercise, place either your pointer fingers or thumbs at point 4—on top of the eye socket one-third of the way in from the outside corners of your eyes (see the following figure). Press and massage for a count of 10 and release. Repeat for a total of three times.

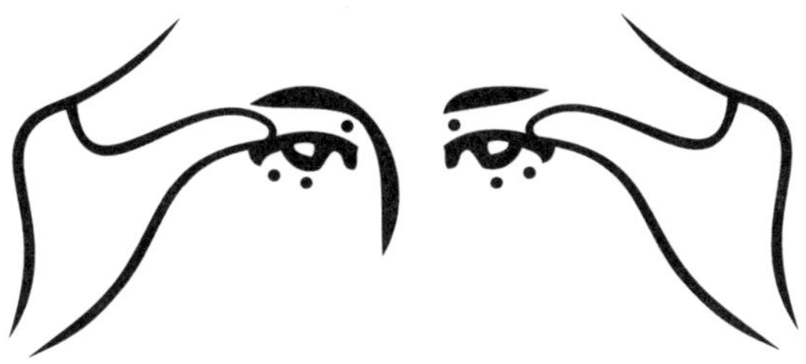

FIGURE 17.
Massaging acupressure point 4.

Next, place either your middle or index fingers at point 5 on your temples by following your eyebrows to their outside edge and then to the soft depressions on the sides of your head (see following figure). Press and massage for a count of 10 and release. Repeat for a total of three times.

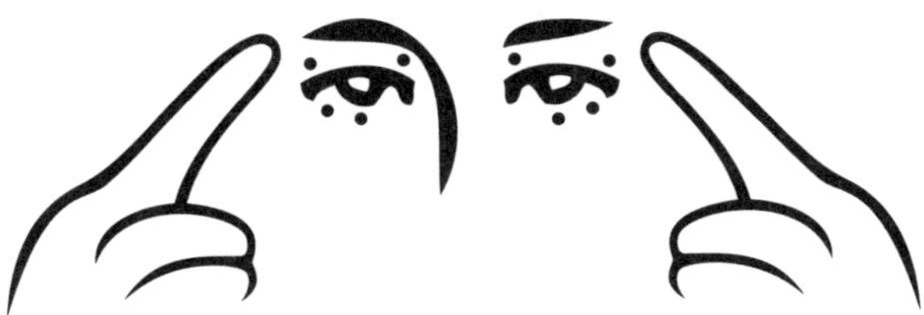

FIGURE 18.
Massaging acupressure point 5.

For the last eye massage, starting at the inside corner of each eye, use your three middle fingers to lightly rub the eye sockets around your eyes (see following figure). Rub in a circular motion—as you circle your eyes, rub in tiny circles with your three fingers. Rub up the bridge of your nose, across your eyebrows, toward your temples, down and back around the lower rims of your eye sockets to your nose again. Do this 10 times, then pause, and then repeat, for a total of three cycles.

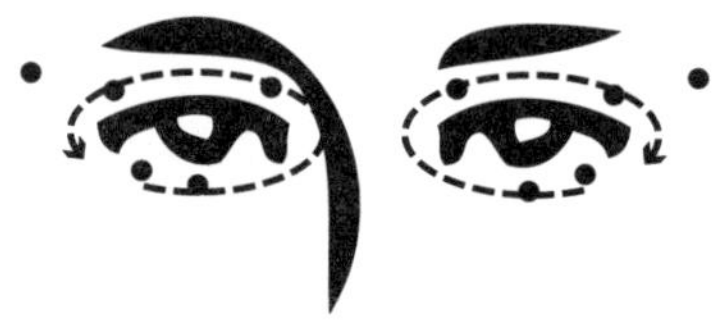

FIGURE 19. Final eye massage.

A few notes on the above exercises:

- Do not rub in the opposite direction, as this will promote weakening of the eye muscles and the formation of wrinkles. In addition, when doing the above massages, always use a healing cream as a lubricant, made of natural ingredients (I recommend Dr. Chang's Royal Jade Cream; see the end of this chapter for purchasing information).
- If you have cataracts or glaucoma, practice the above exercises (as well as the palm rubbing exercise shown) for 20 minutes daily. Whenever your eyes are tired, do all of the eye exercises, as they will revitalize your entire body. Be sure to consult your physician for serious eye conditions such as these as well.
- It is not necessary to put hard pressure on points that are painful. When you come to a painful point, a very light touch will accomplish the goals of the exercise.

After the acupressure exercises, you should perform what I consider to be the most important eye exercise of them all: the palming exercise.

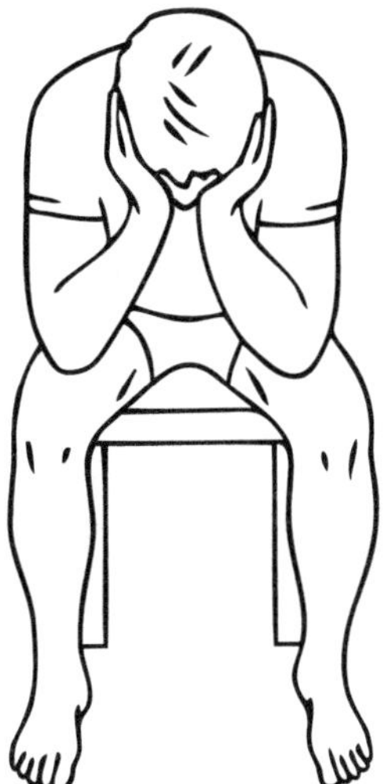

FIGURE 20. Palming exercise for eyes.

Before you begin, always make sure your hands are clean, because you'll be bringing healing energy into your eyes through your hands. When you're ready, rub your hands together briskly for 10 seconds to warm them through friction; rub until they are quite warm. Now, with your full palms over both eyes, cup your hands. I prefer to do this while sitting in a chair, my elbows on my knees and the heels of my palms facing in at the bridge of my nose, resting my head on my palms (see figure above). Hold for a count of eight seconds (do not press your eyes), then release. Repeat the whole process two more times for a total of three times. This exercise will bring a lot of energy and warmth to your eyes. You have a natural instinct in you to do this exercise: it is common sign language for babies to rub their eyes when they are tired and need to sleep, and people continue to do this into adulthood when they are tired. I believe it's the power of the hands to heal through massage, just as when you rub your stomach when it hurts.

The last eye exercise you should perform simply involves looking around. This exercise will strengthen your eyes and the muscles surrounding them. As shown in the following figure, you will be looking around in all directions, toward all of the acupressure points.

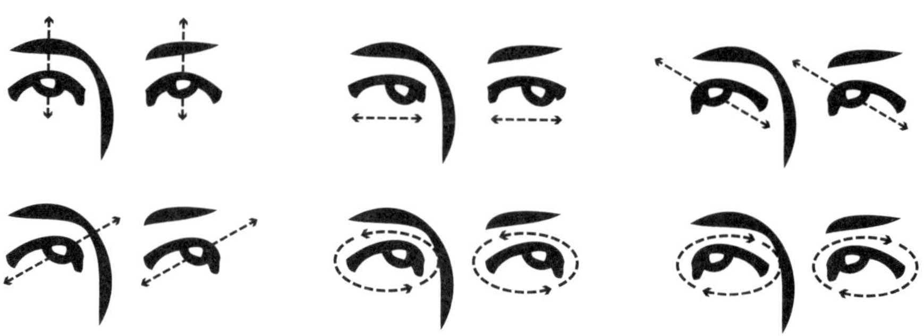

FIGURE 21. Exercise with multiple eye motions.

With your head straight, move your eyes slowly and deliberately. First look up to the ceiling, then down to the floor. Next, look back and forth from the far left to the far right. Now look to the upper right, to the lower left, and back up, and then switch sides. Now rotate your eyes in a clockwise direction, and then counter-clockwise. Finish these exercises by rubbing your palms together and then cupping them over your eyes to bring them warmth and energy.

3. Nose

Next, perform the nose exercises. The nose, sinuses, and lungs are all connected and share an energy flow, so health issues with one will adversely affect the other, and if one is strong it will share its strength with the others. Keeping them all healthy keeps nose-related issues, such as runny nose, blocked sinuses, colds, and allergies, to a minimum. By stimulating three pressure points around your nose, you can keep your nasal and sinus passages healthy, and, indirectly, help keep your lungs healthy as well. Do this throughout the day as needed, or at a minimum once within this complete routine. First, using the tips of your index fingers as shown in the following figure, press down with heavy pressure at the base of your nose. Press for about 10 seconds, and then briefly rub the points.

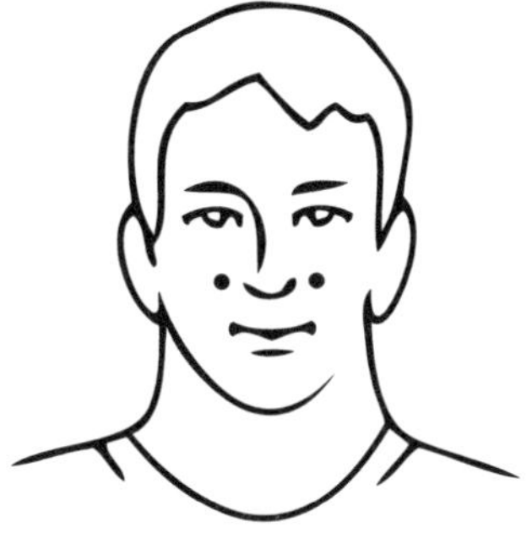
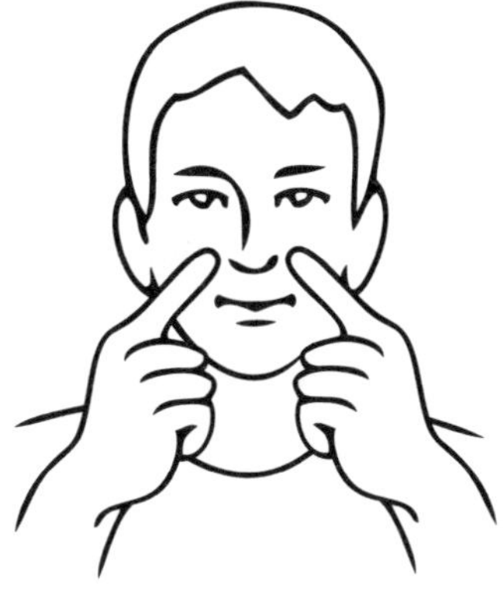

FIGURE 22.
Internal exercise for the nose, first position.

Next, again for about 10 seconds, press the points about halfway up your nose on each side, and then rub briefly (see below).

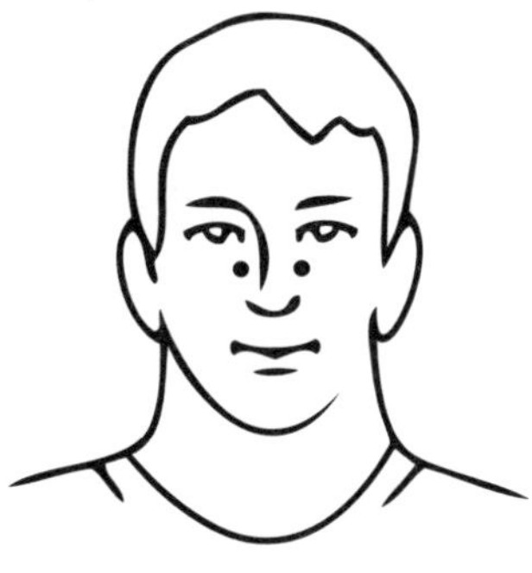
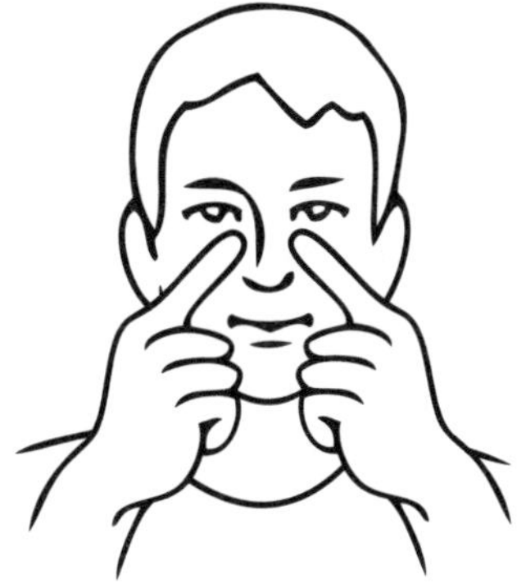

FIGURE 23.
Internal exercise for the nose, second position.

Now press the point midway between your eyebrows with both fingers for about 10 seconds, and again rub briefly.

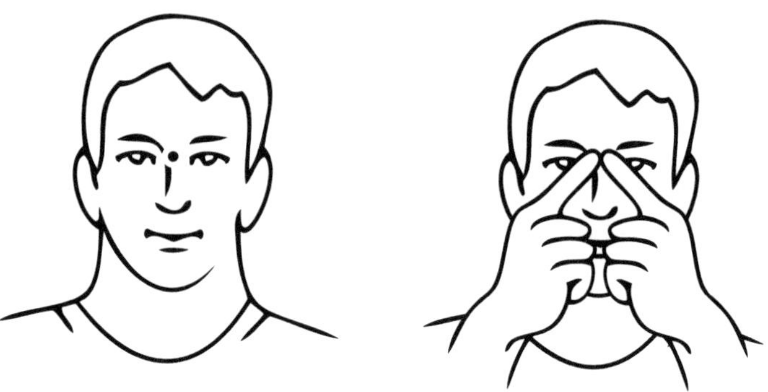

FIGURE 24.
Internal exercise for the nose, third position.

Repeat this whole exercise three times, always starting at the base of your nose and ending at the top. Rub in a continual, flowing motion. As I mentioned, the pressure should be a deep, penetrating pressure. You may find the points to be sensitive or painful in the beginning, which indicates a weakened or blocked energy flow. If you continue to perform this exercise every day, the pain will subside over time.

4. Ears

Your ears never rest, be it daytime or nighttime. Even while you are sleeping your ears are always receiving stimuli. The following exercise is the Taoist way of both stimulating and giving rest to the ears. It is their belief that this exercise helps protect hearing into old age, as well as wards off ear-related ailments such as ringing of the ears. The following exercise should be performed in its entirety at least once a day, and more if you are experiencing ear problems.

First, place both index fingers behind your upper ears, and fold your upper ears over such that they seal off the opening of your ear canal from sound (or by pressing down on the flap over the ear canal). Now, while holding your ear canal closed, use your middle fingers to tap the fingernails on your index fingers. If you are doing it correctly you will hear a metallic sound similar to the beating of a drum, which is known as "beating the heavenly drum." Slowly tap out a regular rhythm 12 to 36 times. Pause, then repeat, then pause and repeat.

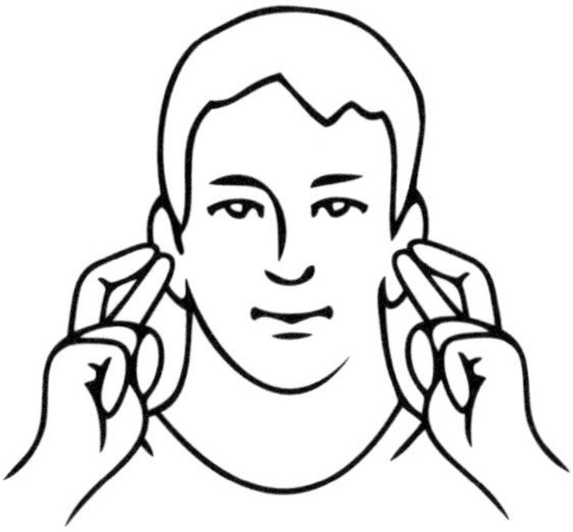

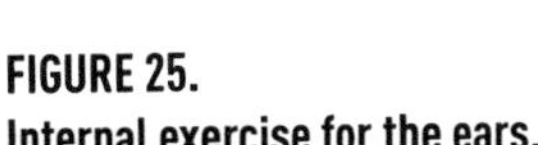

FIGURE 25.
Internal exercise for the ears.

5. Mouth

The following exercises will help you keep your mouth, teeth, and gums in top condition throughout your lifetime.

Tongue and Saliva Exercise

Saliva helps prevent tooth decay, aids in digestion, and possesses natural healing powers. Use the germ-killing ability of saliva to cleanse your mouth. This exercise may be done after meals, upon waking to remove bad breath, and at other appropriate times.

1. Roll your tongue around the inside of your mouth and across your gums and teeth. Use your tongue as you would a toothbrush.

2. As you roll your tongue around your mouth, your salivary glands will excrete saliva. Do not swallow it, but allow it to collect until you have a mouthful.
3. Swish the saliva around as if you were using a mouthwash. Wash the entire inside of your mouth including your gums and in between your teeth.
4. Divide the saliva into three equal parts and swallow each part separately and slowly until your mouth is clear.

Tongue Exercise #2

This exercise is wonderful for strengthening your tongue muscle. Stick your tongue out and down as far as it can go as shown in the figure, and hold it there for four seconds, opening your eyes wide while you do it. Pull your tongue back inside your mouth and pause, then repeat the exercise two more times.

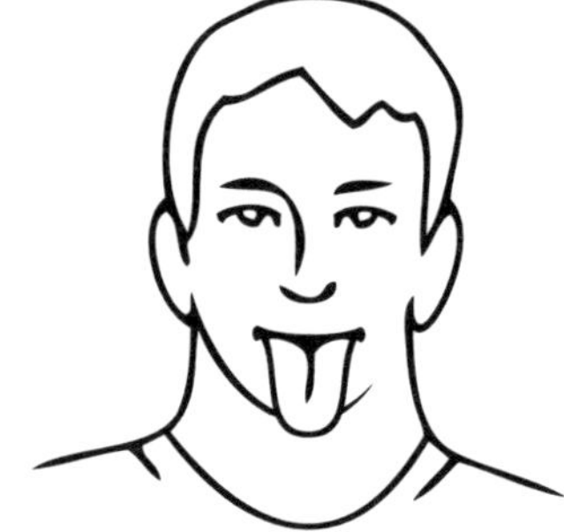

FIGURE 26.
Tongue exercise.

Gum Pressure Exercise

There are points at the top and bottom of the lips that can be pressed to stimulate the energy meridians that supply the mouth, teeth, and gums. This exercise may be done in the morning, after meals, or whenever appropriate.

Press the points designated in the following figure. Press with a firm and steady pressure and follow with a rubbing movement to energize the area. Repeat three times.

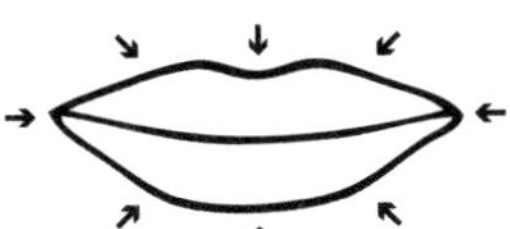

FIGURE 27. Pressure points for the gum exercise.

Teeth Clicking Exercise

You need to protect your teeth from decay. As teeth age they also loosen and need help to stay tight. You want to prevent faulty chewing from developing because chewing is so integral to proper digestion. Once digestion is diminished, a decreased capacity to absorb nutritive elements from food develops, which leads to a generally weakened internal system. This exercise is designed to strengthen and protect the teeth.

Click your teeth together 36 times. Open them about a half-inch each time you click.

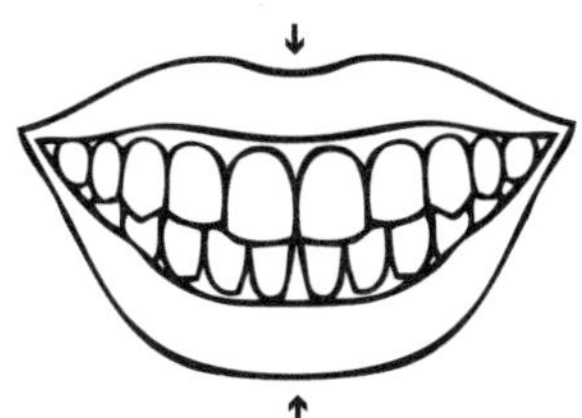

FIGURE 28. Teeth clicking exercise.

When practiced in the morning this exercise will help awaken you; when done during the day, it will help keep your mind alert. Clicking or clenching your teeth during more immunologically vulnerable times such as sexual intercourse, orgasm, or moving the bowels helps protect your body and keep up your natural defenses.

6. Neck and Thyroid

The neck connects the brain to the rest of the body, both in nerve impulses and energy, so it is an important part to exercise. This first exercise strengthens that connection, as well as offers aesthetic benefits by helping prevent a double chin or helping firm one if you already have one. First look straight ahead, not tilting your head up, down, or to the side. Now lift your head and hold a firm, extended stretch for four seconds, as if straining to look at something in the sky (your jaw should be further out than the top of your mouth, as in the following figure), then relax and look straight ahead. Pause briefly, and repeat two more times. Now do the same exercise, except instead of looking up, look up and to the right, and repeat a total of three times; then look up and to the left, repeating a total of three times.

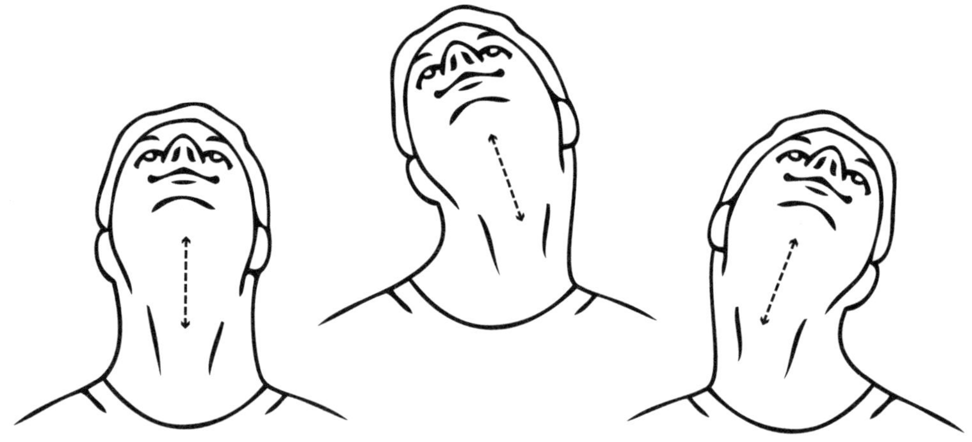

FIGURE 29. Neck exercises: looking up, up right, and up left.

The thyroid gland controls our metabolism. Massaging your thyroid sends energy into the area to help the thyroid function normally. Your metabolism will be improved, thus boosting the breakdown of food and aiding digestion and absorption of nutrients. Massage will also help your body eliminate more poisons and toxins. If you have a thyroid condition, it may help to the point that thyroid medication is unnecessary (of course, consult with your doctor before adjusting your own prescription).

The acupressure points are designated in the following figure. Contact these spots when you are performing the massage. The figure on the right shows the hand position for the massage. First massage the front and back of your neck, then hold each point firmly for four seconds each.

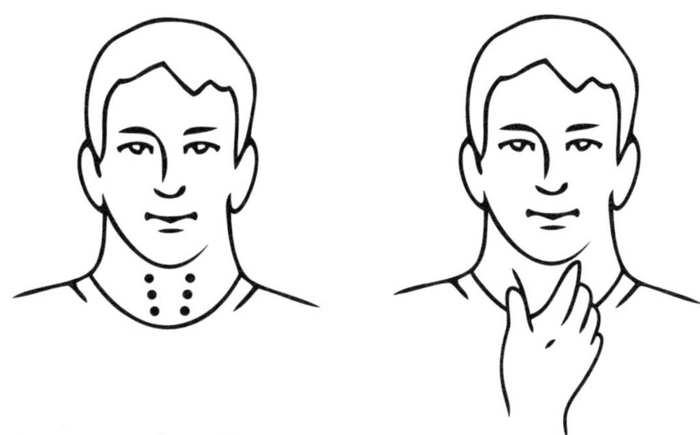

FIGURE 30. Acupressure points and the internal exercise for the thyroid.

7. Lungs

The internal exercises for the lungs strengthen the entire respiratory system. They also help heal illnesses related to the lungs, such as colds.

To measure the health of your lungs, focus on the length of time it takes you to inhale and then to exhale. If the time it takes you to exhale is longer than the time it takes you to inhale, ill health is indicated, since more is going out than coming in. On the other hand, if the reverse is true, that's a healthy sign, as more energy is being taken in.

To perform the lung exercises, stand with your feet parallel to each other and shoulder-width apart. Keep your back straight, hold your head up straight with your chin slightly toward your chest, and stretch your neck upward. Now clasp your hands behind your back as shown in the following figure and exhale all of the air from your lungs.

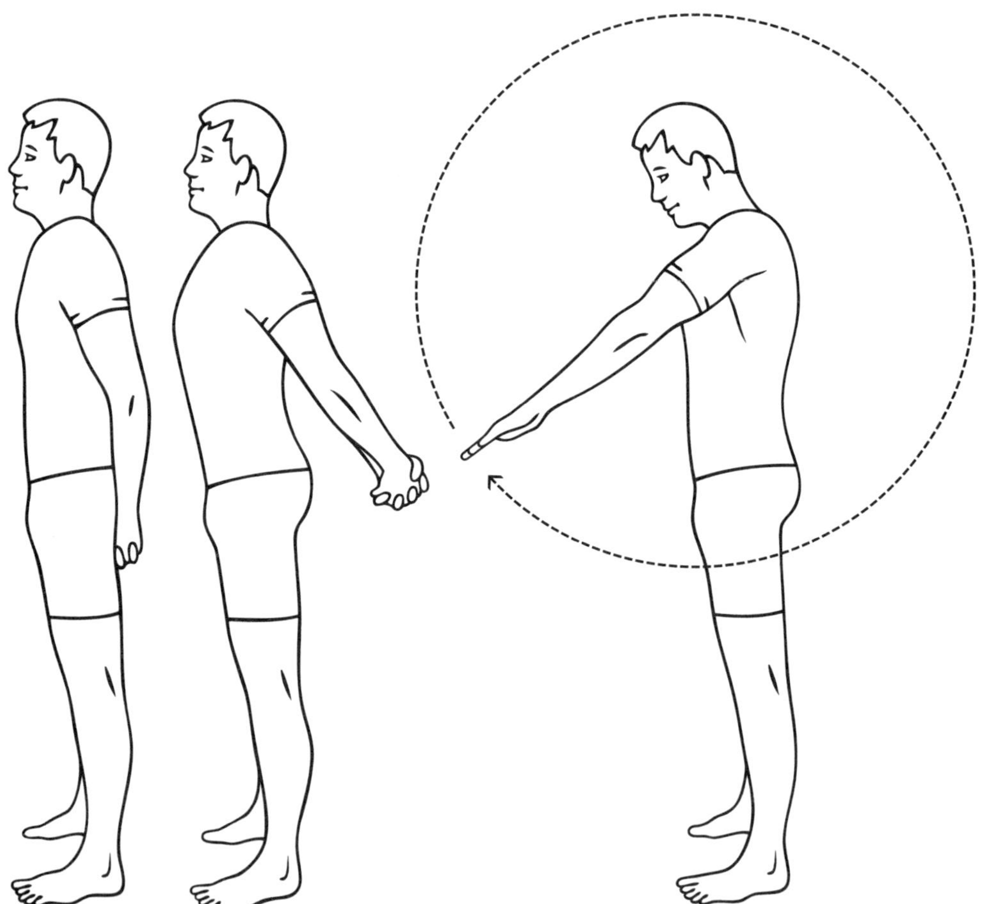

FIGURE 31. Internal exercise for the lungs.

When the air is out, begin inhaling slowly, expanding your lungs while pushing your hands away from your back (see figure). As you do this, keep your body still with your chin tucked into your chest; use your chest only to breathe during the exercise. Experience the fresh energy coming into your lungs and invigorating the tissues.

Now drop your arms and begin exhaling; hold your arms out in front of you with your fingers pointed, and then raise them over your head. Circle them behind your back and then back to the front of your body, as shown in the following figure. As you exhale, feel the stale air, toxins, and germs exit your lungs.

Now lock your fingers behind your back and begin the first exercise again, performing another complete cycle.

8. Heart

There is no rest for our heart. It is one of the first functioning organs in the womb and beats our entire lives until our death, so we obviously need to pay very close attention to its health. The following exercises are for strengthening the heart and its surrounding blood vessels. Practicing them regularly may help prevent and heal diseases and problems of the heart.

Heart Massage

This exercise is best performed standing. First rub your hands together vigorously to get the energy flowing into your palms and fingers. Now place your palms over your heart, which in most people is under and protruding to the left of their sternum. Rub up and down and in a circular motion over this area. To be clear you are not literally massaging the heart itself, but channeling warmth and good, healthy energy to it. Continue rubbing in a small, circular motion down your left arm.

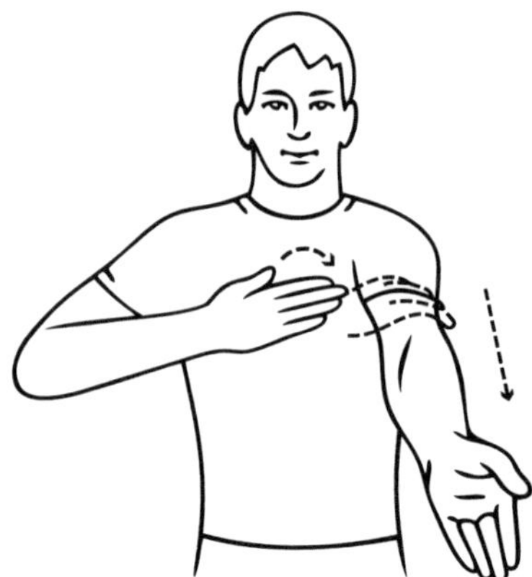

FIGURE 32. Heart massage.

9. Stomach

You may sit, stand, or lie down for this exercise. Rub your hands vigorously until they are quite warm. Then rub your stomach in a circular motion, feeling the energy move from your palms to your stomach.

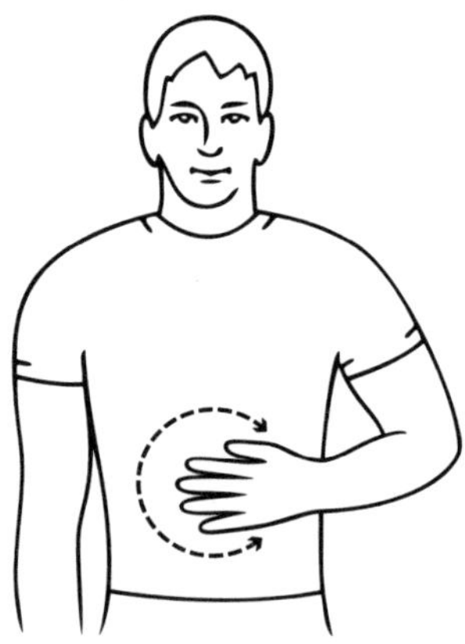

FIGURE 33. Stomach healing exercise.

See the end of the liver section for an additional exercise that benefits the stomach.

10. Liver

The three main filters of the body are the heart, kidneys, and liver. Liver exercises are very important because the liver filters toxins from our bodies. Practice this exercise every morning to help keep your liver functioning properly.

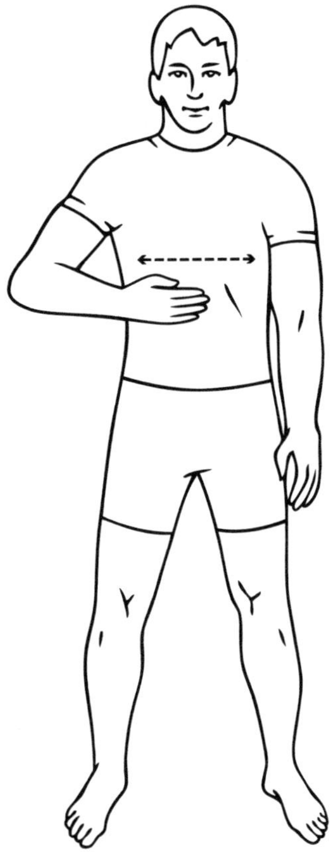

FIGURE 34. Internal exercise for the liver.

Sit or lie down in a comfortable position. Your liver lies just under the right rib cage, so begin by rubbing over your liver and then moving across your chest to the left. This will stimulate energy and blood flow to the liver. Place the palm of your right hand on the right side of your body just at the base of your rib cage as shown in the preceding figure. Press the heel of your hand along your chest, following the line of your lower rib bones. Rub toward your sternum (in the middle) and then over to the left side. Rubbing once from right to left equals one round; repeat 36 rounds total.

You can also perform this exercise from left to right (with your left hand) to strengthen your stomach, which lies below the left side of the chest. Exercising both sides will strengthen your digestive system, since those two organs are related, and encourage smooth functioning between them.

11. Kidneys

This exercise will stimulate, energize, strengthen, and heal your kidneys and related adrenal glands, located directly behind the small of your back. You should perform this every morning and whenever you experience back pain.

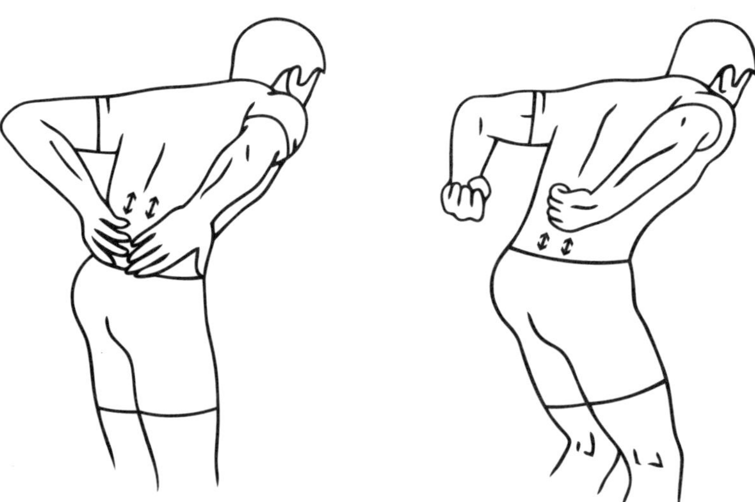

FIGURE 35. Internal exercises for the kidneys.

This exercise is best performed standing. First rub your hands together vigorously to get the energy flowing into your palms and fingers. Now place your palms on the small of your back, keeping your body tilted slightly forward, as shown in the preceding figure. Feel the energy and heat flowing from your hands into your back, kidneys, and adrenal glands.

Massage the small of your back by rubbing up and down, and then by rubbing in a circular motion, across your back. Next, clench your fists and gently pound the small of your back for a few seconds with the back of your hands (see figure). Repeat the rubbing and pounding exercises for a total of three times.

12. Arms

I believe that energy circulates throughout the body along microscopic pathways called meridians. While this has been a part of Taoist beliefs for thousands of years, in the past century scientific evidence that supports these ideas has emerged.

Meridians are symmetrical bilateral channels that range between 20 and 50 millimicrons across. They have thin membranes surrounding them and are filled with a transparent fluid. The places at which the branches reach the skin's surface are the acupressure points mentioned throughout this book.

Because of the meridian connections, you may use the arm massage to stimulate your heart, lungs, and intestines.

First, stretch your right arm out, palm up. Place your left palm on the inside of your right shoulder (see following figure). Now firmly rub your palm down through the inside of your elbow to your fingers in one continuous motion. Next, stretch your arm out, palm down. Rub your left palm over the top of your arm, up to the shoulder. Repeat the above two steps 12 times, then switch arms and do it on the other side.

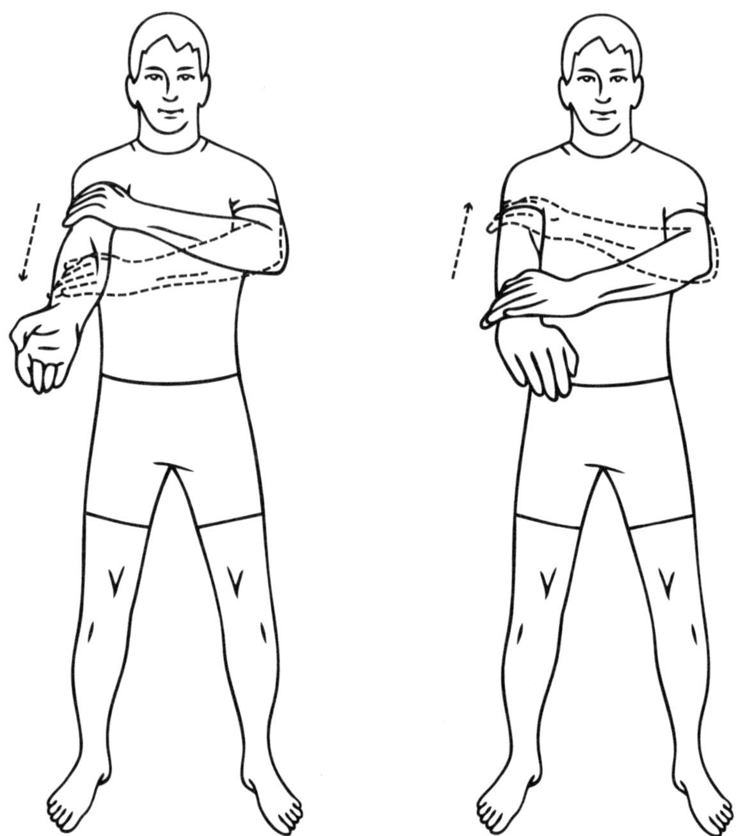

FIGURE 36. Downward and upward arm rubbing.

13. Legs

For a review of meridians, please see the previous section on arm rubbing (number 12).

Due to the gravitational pull on the circulatory system, blood tends to pool in the feet and legs, especially with age. By stimulating the meridians of the leg, you can strengthen the healthy flow of blood, thus helping prevent blood from accumulating there and hampering your circulatory system.

Upwardly massaging the inside of your legs will stimulate the blood circulation in the lower half of your body. This exercise can be done standing, sitting, or lying down. First place the palms of your hands on the inside of your legs, at the ankles. Slowly slide your palms up your legs, through the inside of your knees up to the crotch. Keep the pressure firm enough so you feel a slight warmth in your legs as you massage them. Repeat 12 times. Keep in mind that you should be breathing normally throughout the exercise. The most important part of this exercise is the massage of the knee to the thigh, so much so that you could just focus on this part and still achieve most of the benefit. Also note that morning is a good time to perform this exercise, as it will energize your body.

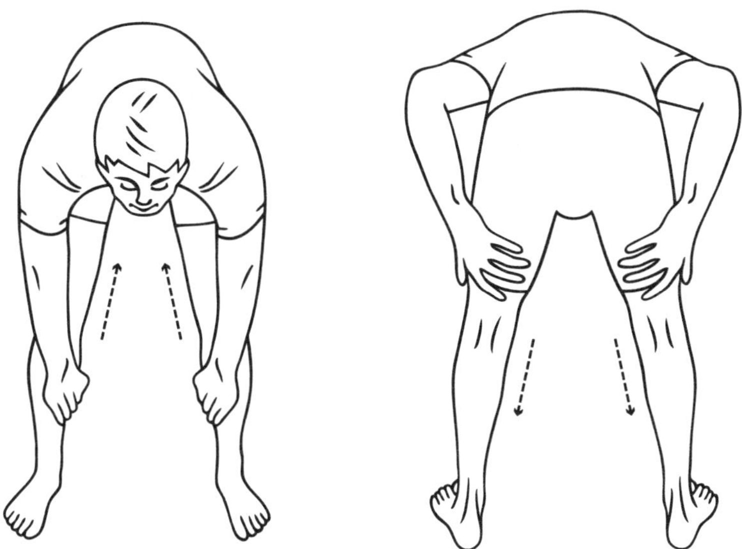

FIGURE 37. Upward and downward leg massage.

By massaging your legs on the outside in a downward motion, you are helping dispel energy from your body as well as improving or preventing such conditions as high blood pressure, water retention, and obesity. This exercise can also be done standing, sitting, or lying down. First place your palms on the outside of your thighs. In one continuous motion, slide your hands down your legs along the outside of your knees and calves, down to your ankles (see figure). Repeat 12 times, breathing normally. It is not recommended that you perform this exercise in the morning since it helps move energy out of your body.

14. Head Hanging

The head hanging exercise is a great one to really relax your upper body. It focuses on the muscles responsible for the most frequent forms of nervous and muscular tension—the region of the upper spine, neck, and shoulders. This area is very sensitive to stress-induced tension, and when stressed it causes blockage of blood and energy circulation to the head. In addition, vital nerves can be pinched between the head and body when tense. People who experience chronic stress and nervous tension, especially those who are affected physically with hunched shoulders, cramps, and so on, will benefit tremendously by practicing this exercise once or twice a day.

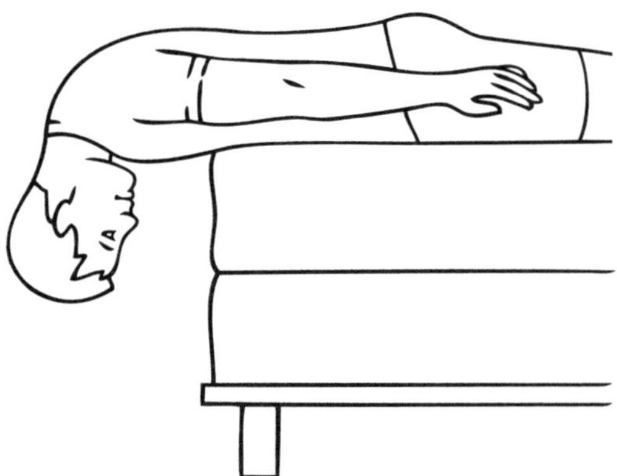

FIGURE 38. The head hang.

In comfortable clothes, lie stomach-down on a table or flat space off the floor such that your head can hang freely from your shoulders (see preceding figure). Keep your arms extended flat to your sides and let your head hang down completely, heavy and relaxed. Lie in this position for a while, letting your neck and shoulder muscles stretch and letting gravity do its job to bring the head further down. Breathe slowly and naturally without straining. Hold for four seconds, and repeat if desired.

If you feel strained or want to pause in between hanging your head, lay your hands on the floor as shown in the next figure. Continue to focus on breathing deeply and steadily.

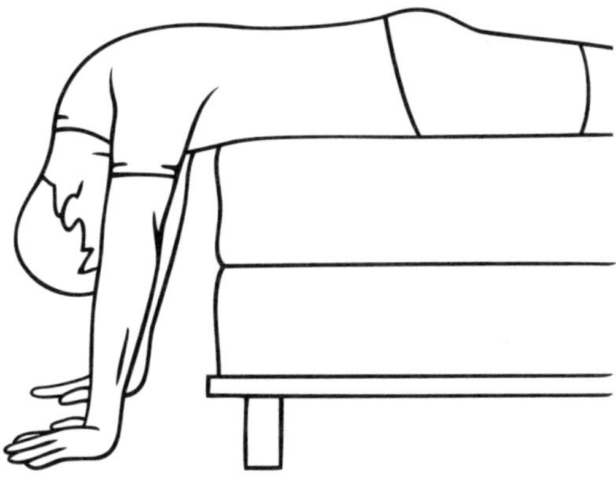

FIGURE 39. A variation of the head hang.

15. Internal Organ Relaxation

Our ancestors from long, long ago did not walk upright, and our circulatory system has not quite caught up with our evolution. As opposed to humans, who have gravity pressing down on their piled-up internal organs to compact them, the organs of our four-legged ancestors hung freely in their abdomen. The stance of four-legged creatures allows for the proper amount of circulation and blood. We need to give our internal organs a break and let them relax as nature truly intended.

Get in the position of a four-legged animal such as a dog. As in the following figure, get on your hands, knees, and toes. Look forward and keep your chest parallel to the floor. Now pause a moment to allow blood to circulate freely into and around all of your internal organs; focus on this and feel it happening. Blood is being retained in your stomach and the intestines to strengthen digestion and elimination. Breathe easily and naturally; you may synchronize your breathing with the movements of the exercise if you wish, but it's not necessary.

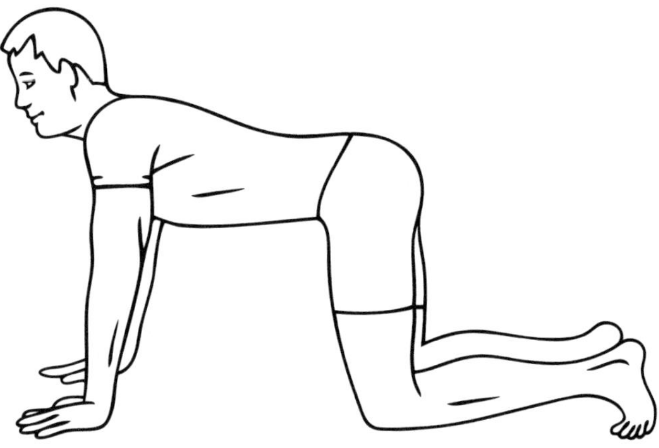

FIGURE 40. Internal organ relaxation.

Now slowly sit back on your heels and lower your forehead to the floor. Close your eyes and stretch your arms out in front of you as shown on the following page. Keep this position for a few seconds, and then come back to the kneeling position. Repeat this cycle seven times.

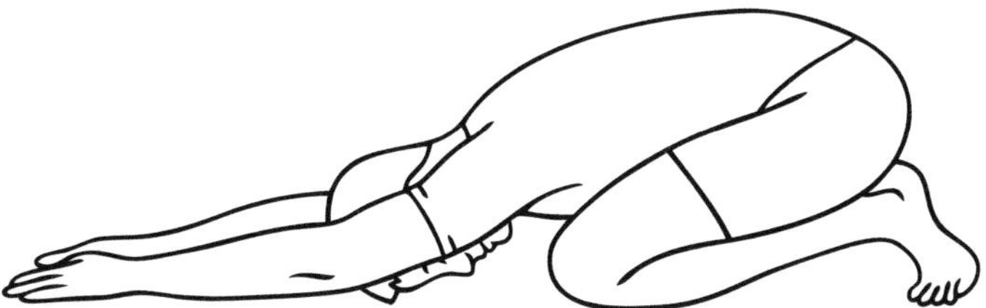

FIGURE 41. Blood is flowing to the heart, lungs, and brain in this position.

When you rest on your heels, blood is forced to flow to your heart, lungs, and brain. Blood is then easily returned to your heart as well, giving it a chance to rest and not work so hard. I recommend you do this every morning. It's an excellent, soothing way to complete your internal exercise routine. Furthermore, because blood flow to the brain is reduced during sound sleep, this exercise will bring blood to your brain, helping you feel fresh, alert, alive, and ready to start your day.

The Taoists believed that if the body's ultimate natural state was achieved through all of these exercises that it would lead to eternal life. They also recognized that not everyone could achieve this perfect state of their body, but that it should be something everyone is continually striving for and working toward. They felt that one could at least live a pain-free life and be utterly happy.

For more information on the internal exercises and products mentioned in this chapter, go to:
www.DOITORAGEQUICKLY.com
www.JBBERNS.com

4
MOUTH HEALTH

For 60 Seconds:
Use remarkable peelu bark to brush your teeth, and don't forget your internal exercises of the mouth.

This chapter addresses exercises and actions you can take to keep your mouth, teeth, and gums in top condition throughout your lifetime.

Internal Exercises for the Mouth

In Chapter 3, Internal Exercises, there is a section of mouth exercises designed to strengthen the mouth muscles, prevent tooth decay, and protect and heal the teeth and gums. The exercises are aligned with Taoist and Hindu principles and show you how to stimulate all aspects of your mouth to keep it healthy and strong. I highly recommend going through them every day as part of your internal exercises routine.

Peelu Bark

Oh peelu, oh peelu, I love you. Why am I singing the praises of a tree bark that grows in India? Please let me explain. As all my family and friends know, I have been brushing my teeth with peelu bark for well over a decade. A number of those friends are dentists, and I have never needed to see them as a patient since I've known them. I don't get cavities—the last time I did was when I was still a child. In general the people of India have extraordinarily healthy teeth as well, particularly given the economic circumstances of many of its citizens.

For centuries, people of Asia, Africa, and the Middle East have cleaned their teeth by chewing the dried branches of the Peelu tree. They continue to this day because even compared to modern dentistry techniques, it is still highly effective in preventing cavities, maintaining healthy gums, and keeping teeth white. The Peelu tree (botanical name: *Salvadora persica*) has been studied to understand why it is so effective:

- Peelu sticks contain gentle yet effective fibers that softly scrub teeth.
- It contains a natural chlorine that whitens and removes tartar and stains (tartar is a residue that yellows the teeth).
- It contains tannic acid and vitamin C, making it beneficial for healthy gums.
- It contains sulfur, which helps keep the mouth clean.

In contrast, commercial toothpastes tend to have harsh abrasives that over the years strip the thin top layer of enamel away. Enamel is white in color, but the dentin layer below it is yellow, which becomes more exposed and accounts for most people's teeth yellowing as they age. Enamel also helps protect our teeth, and as it thins our teeth are much more sensitive to heat and cold. Peelu is an excellent solution because it whitens while it protects the enamel.

I use the fibers of peelu, the actual bark ground into a powder, because it's the most effective. However, peelu is now made into an all-natural toothpaste as well (see figure), which is a good alternative if someone doesn't like the texture of the bark. Swish it in your mouth for 60 seconds after you're done brushing your teeth. It's also a great idea to use a towel to buff your teeth to a shine after brushing with peelu, especially the front four or five teeth. Now go smile in the mirror!

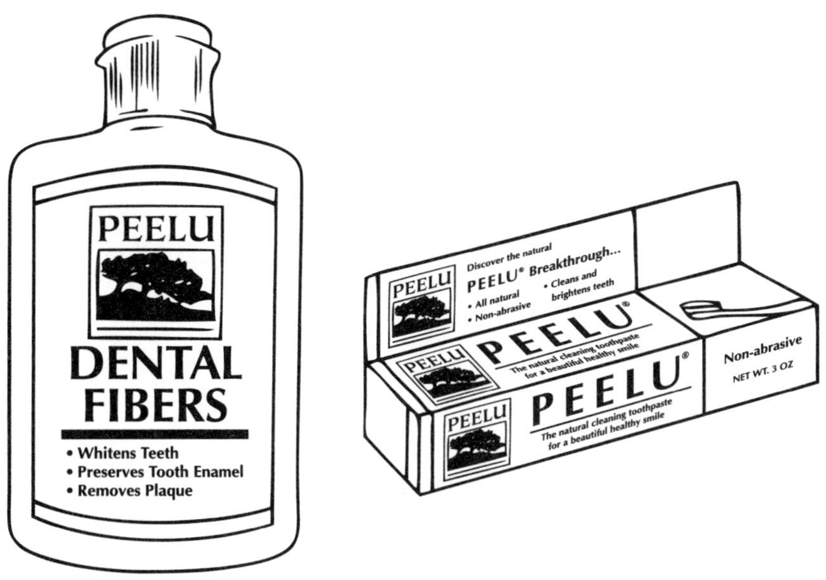

FIGURE 42. Peelu dental fibers and peelu toothpaste.

I can't say enough about the wonders of peelu bark. It makes your teeth look great and keeps them in great shape. It might even save you some money, be it in dental supplies or dental bills.

Attend to your mouth, teeth, and gums with tender loving care. They will feel great, and you'll preserve your teeth for your lifetime.

For more information on where to buy peelu bark and related products, go to:
www.DOITORAGEQUICKLY.com
www.JBBERNS.com

5
LOOFAH MASSAGE

For 60 Seconds:
Massage yourself with a loofah sponge.

The loofah plant is a year-round climbing plant, related to both gourds and cucumbers, and thrives in warm, dry climates. It produces cylindrical fruits, and as it ripens, its interior is transformed into a spongy fibrous mass similar to mesh. The fruit is then harvested and the outer skin is removed. After this the fruit is dried and the seeds are shaken out, and this remaining mass is what makes up the material to produce a loofah sponge.

Because of its coarse texture and absorbency when wet, the loofah plant has been used in bathing for centuries. When used to gently scrub the skin, the loofah exfoliates the skin, removing the rough outermost layer and leaving clean pores and soft, smooth skin. It also stimulates surface blood circulation.

Even more important, I believe, is using the loofah to give yourself a massage while showering. In order to do this, you should purchase a loofah sponge in the shape of a glove. Another option, which achieves the same effect, is a sisal glove. I recommend the Sisal Bath Glove by Swissco. See the end of this chapter for purchasing information.

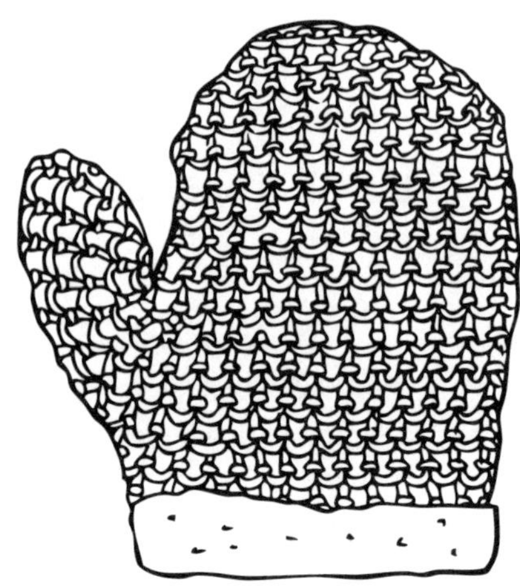

FIGURE 43. A sisal glove for exfoliation massage (it has the same effect as a loofah sponge).

I recommend using the loofah as a massage tool because you can essentially multitask in the shower: you'll remove dead skin cells, invigorate blood circulation, and massage the lymphatic system to help remove toxins from your body all at the same time.

To understand the importance of stimulating the lymphatic system, let me first give you a brief explanation of what the lymphatic system does. It is made up of lymph nodes, organs, and ducts. The lymph nodes are clustered throughout the body and connected by an extensive network of lymphatic vessels, which act as the immune system's circulatory system. The lymphatic system transports a clear, watery fluid called lymph. One of the lymphatic system's most important functions is to distribute immune cells and other factors throughout the body. It also interacts with the blood circulatory system to drain fluid from cells and tissues. In addition, the lymphatic system transports microorganisms, other foreign substances, cancer cells, and dead or damaged cells from the tissues to the lymph nodes and then to the bloodstream.

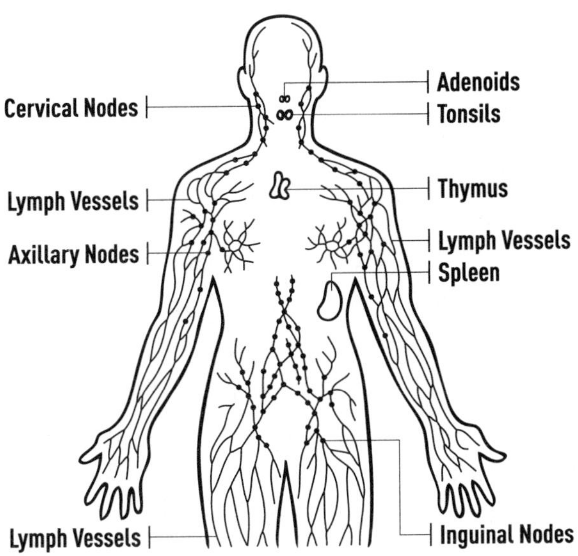

FIGURE 44. The lymphatic system.

The lymphatic system does not have a pump for lymph as the circulatory system does for blood, however. Rather, the transport of lymph is due to breathing movements and skeletal muscle contractions, and it moves in only one direction due to a large number of valves that impose a one-way flow. Massaging the body's soft tissues will also help move lymph through the system.

To give you an example of how the loofah massage benefits the lymphatic system, let me tell you about an old injury I have been managing. I have meniscus tears on both of my knees that I have chosen not to have surgically repaired. Because of this, after I finish my yoga or martial arts routines, my knees usually begin to swell. I then immediately jump into the shower and use the loofah glove for one minute on my entire body. If I am pressed for time I start with my knees and work up to my neck. The loofah glove helps move the stagnated lymph that accumulates around both of my knees, and after just 60 seconds of massage I have better range of motion and less swelling in my knees. It's incredible.

Lymphatic massage utilizes pressure combined with soft pumping movements in the direction of the lymph nodes. You must push down firmly. Use the glove with water only—the sensation is refreshing, and your skin will feel tingly during the massage. If you are uncomfortable with the tingling sensation and the loofah feels too rough, add soap to the glove to lessen the friction. I recommend starting the massage at your ankles and moving up your body. Rub in an up-and-down vertical motion on your lower body, except for your knees, which you should scrub in a circular motion (see figure below).

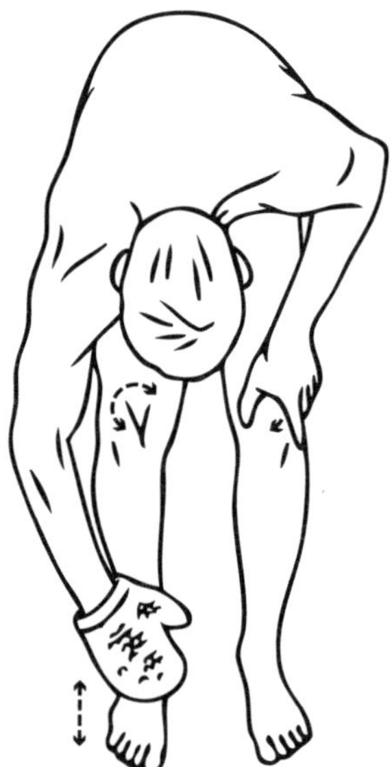

FIGURE 45.
Beginning the exfoliating loofah massage.

Working up your body, scrub your torso in the manner shown in the following figure. Include the full length of your arms (in an up-and-down motion), abdomen (circular motion), and chest (circular motion).

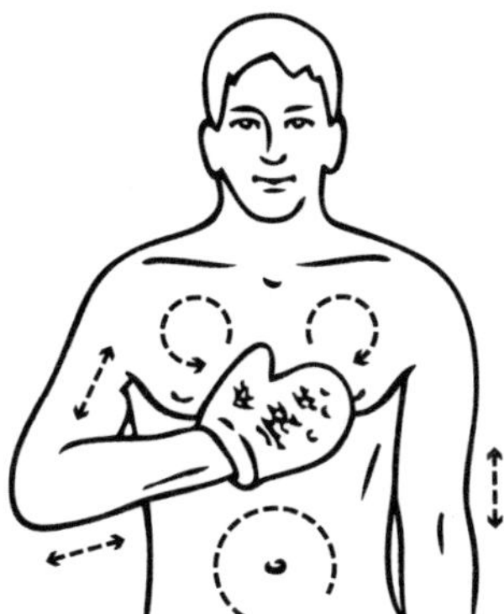

FIGURE 46.
Scrubbing motion on torso during loofah massage.

Be sure to include your back as well. Rub in a vertical motion everywhere but your shoulders, where you should scrub in a circular motion.

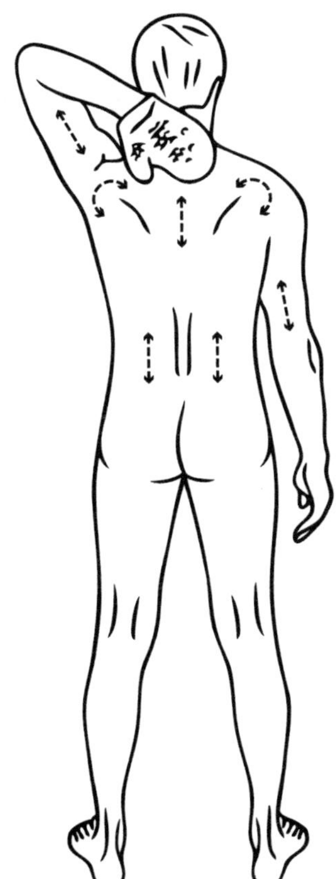

FIGURE 47.
Scrubbing motion on the backside during the shower.

I have been using the loofah glove for many years and I can tell you only wonderful things about the results I have experienced. I even travel with it wherever I go. It is my opinion that not only can immune system function be significantly increased—improving your metabolism and helping your body eliminate waste and toxins—but the increased circulation it promotes retards potential varicose veins and combats cellulite. At the very least it will improve the tone of your skin to minimize the appearance of these conditions.

Give yourself an exfoliating loofah massage during your shower for your health and your appearance. It takes just 60 seconds and you will feel great.

For more information on the loofah massage and products, go to:
www.DOITORAGEQUICKLY.com
www.JBBERNS.com

6
ISOMETRIC EXERCISES

For 60 Seconds:
Contract your muscles—calves, quads, hamstrings, buttocks, back, abs, chest, shoulders, triceps, and biceps.

Isometric exercises have been practiced throughout history. In this form of resistance strength training, a participant will use the muscles of his body to exert a force against an immovable object or hold a contracted muscle in a fixed position for a set duration of time. The word "isometric" comes from the Greek word "iso" meaning "same," and "metric" meaning "length," because an isometric contraction refers to the contraction or tightening of a muscle without changing its length (as compared to isotonic contractions in which the joint angle changes and you move your limbs as the muscle contracts).

An interesting study on frog legs in the 1920s illustrates both the physiology and effectiveness of isometric exercises. Conducted not long after World War I, the study was taken up with wounded soldiers in mind. Thousands of injured U.S. soldiers were in hospitals around the country, in need of rehabilitation before they could return to society. Scientists wanted to know how long it would be before complete immobilization caused extensive muscle degeneration and atrophy in the men. No one expected the incredible results they found.

The researchers had taken healthy frogs and tethered one of their legs so that it was completely immobile, while the other leg was allowed free movement. After two weeks the researchers unwrapped the tethered leg to see how much it had atrophied. To their great surprise, not only had it not atrophied, but it had bulked up!

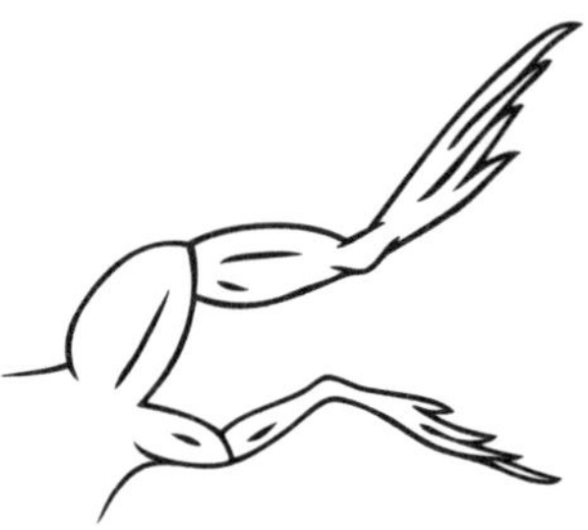

FIGURE 48. The actual illustration for the 1920 frog study is not available, but the dramatization of the results shown here demonstrate the bulked-up immobilized leg (top) versus the normal-size free leg (bottom).

The tethered leg had gotten considerably larger and stronger over the two weeks, to such a degree that the frogs jumped around lopsided because of the disparity of power. In the free leg, as in weight lifting, only a small percentage of muscle fibers were used. However, in the immobilized leg, straining against an immovable bond forced the animals to use every fiber of their muscles over and over. This is the secret of isometric exercises, but no one understood that yet.

The frog experiment was viewed as a failure and exiled to dusty medical book shelving. It didn't have the results the researchers were expecting, and they didn't extrapolate the great application it had to human beings. About 25 years later, after the Second World War, thousands of wounded soldiers again needed to be rehabilitated, and scientists wanted to help them. This time there had been many examples of athletes and circus strongmen since the 1920s who claimed that isometric exercise was the key to superior health, so they were actually looking to confirm results like those found with the frog experiment.

One experiment similar to the frog experiment was done in 1946. Researchers selected 50 healthy men aged 19 to 55 and completely immobilized one of their arms in a plastic cast. The arm was taken out of the cast once a day, whereupon isometric exercises were performed for less than one minute. Once completed, the arm was placed back into the cast. This went on for four weeks. The result? A dramatic increase in strength of the immobilized arm. This time the results were embraced by the medical community and were circulated far and wide. Many other experiments were being done around this time that investigated isometrics and confirmed the frog and cast results. Isometrics came to be thought of as the best, safest, most efficient, and least expensive method of physical rehabilitation known. Not only did the researchers help the wounded soldiers this time, the applications of the research were broadened to help medical patients such as polio victims and athletes with sports injuries.

By the 1960s isometric training had become a popular method of strength training for weight lifters and athletes alike. Celebrity athletes like Micky Mantle and Bruce Lee utilized it. Books on the market brought it to a mass audience, and people across America began performing these exercises for bulk, strength, and endurance. Many different regimens were devised of varying repetition and length. Some even proposed "aerobic isometrics," where one would hold a contraction for several minutes.

In my opinion, the best way to perform isometric exercise is for only seconds at a time. In general, my belief about exercise is that people do it too much. It is not the quantity but the quality of exercise you do, and the consistency in which you perform it, that is necessary for superior results. If you overexercise, you also overwork your organs and musculoskeletal system. Therefore, I believe that the ideal external exercise system will take you just one minute a day (although you can do it throughout the day for one minute at a time). I describe the 10 best exercises below. With these 10 exercises, every major and minor muscle group is addressed and focused upon separately. I have been doing these exercises for over 20 years for just a minute a day and have never aggressively lifted a weight, yet my muscle tone is very well defined.

I recommend the following isometric exercises for overall resistance training for both men and women. Your skin and muscles will feel tight and firm immediately afterward, with little if any jarring effect to your body. In fact, part of what makes these exercises so wonderful is that they cause no stress to joints and muscles. The squeezing effect of the different muscle groups is the best known resistance training I have ever experienced personally, and my past clients experienced amazing results as well.

Below is my list of isometric exercises that you should perform every day (instructions and diagrams to follow).

1. Calves
2. Quadriceps
3. Hamstrings
4. Buttocks
5. Back
6. Abdominals
7. Chest
8. Shoulders
9. Triceps
10. Biceps

The Isometric Exercises

For every contraction you do, focus on and visualize the particular muscle you are squeezing.

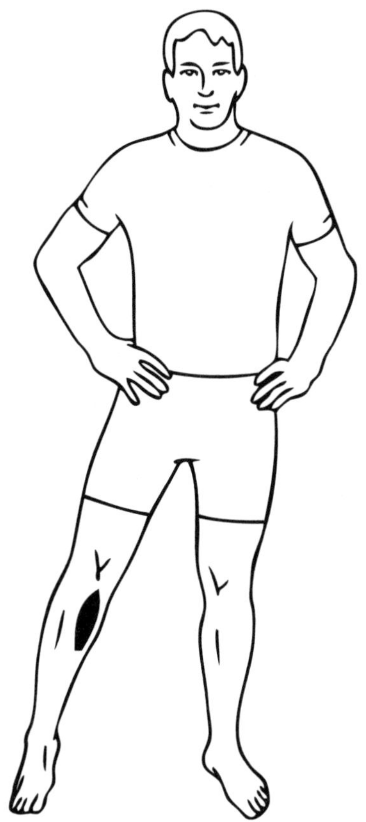

FIGURE 49. Exercise for the calves.

1. Calves

Stand with your legs hip-distance apart. Shift your body to the right side and raise your left foot so it's resting on the ball of the foot. Squeeze your calf for 4 seconds. Next, flatten your foot, and do the same on the other side.

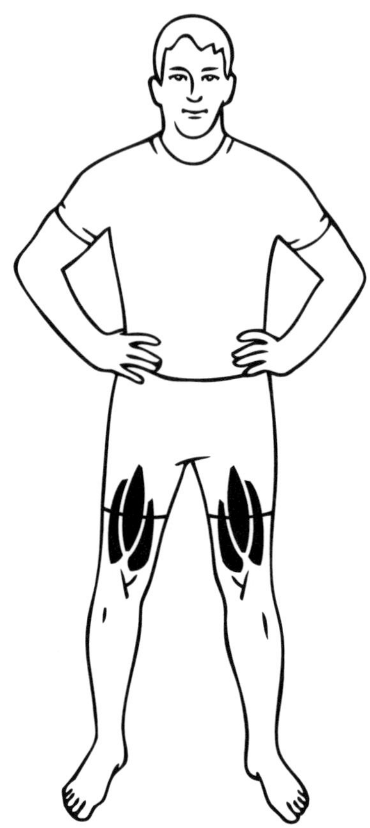

FIGURE 50. Exercise for the quadriceps.

2. Quadriceps

Your quadriceps are the muscles on the front of your upper thighs. Stand with your legs hip-distance apart and squeeze both of your quadriceps for 4 seconds. Repeat, again for 4 seconds.

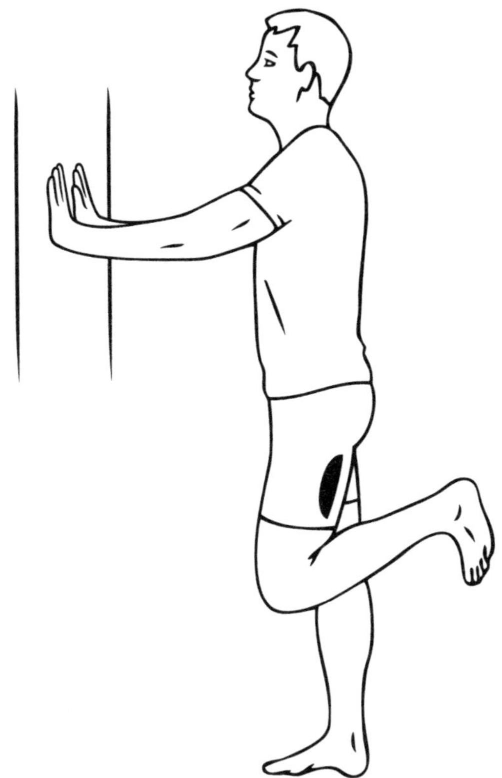

FIGURE 51. Exercise for the hamstrings.

3. Hamstrings

Your hamstrings are the muscles on the backs of your upper legs. Stand with your legs hip-distance apart and rest your hands on a flat surface such as a wall or shower door (if you are in the shower). Bring your right heel up, close to your buttocks, and squeeze your hamstring for 4 seconds. Repeat on the left side. Then repeat one more set on each side for 4 seconds each.

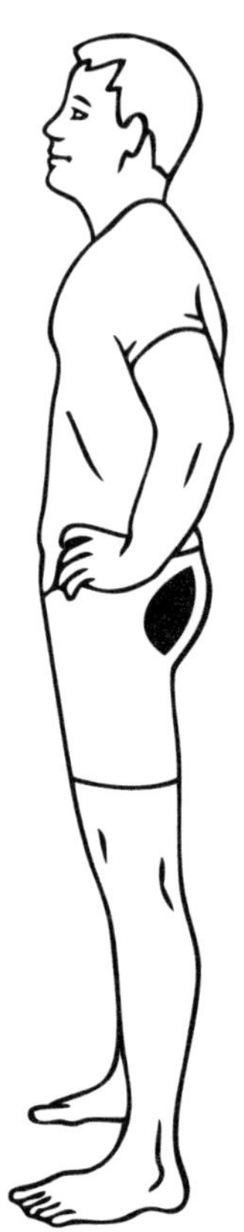

FIGURE 52. Exercise for the buttocks.

4. Buttocks

Squeeze your buttocks for 8 seconds. Try to do this exercise several times a day.

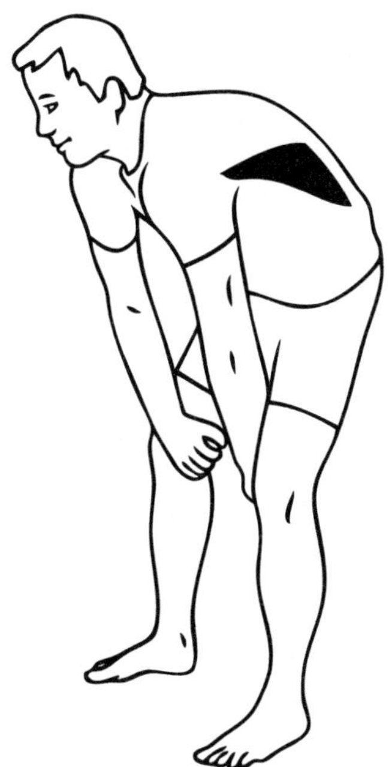

FIGURE 53. Exercise for the back.

5. Back

Stand with your legs hip-distance apart. Bend both legs slightly, and lean forward. Place your hands on the insides of both legs just above your knee, and pull up for 4 seconds. Now rest for 4 seconds, and then repeat the pulling movement for an additional 4 seconds.

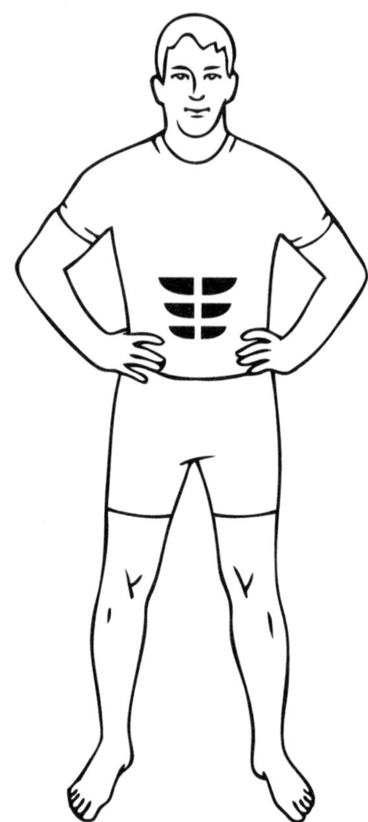

FIGURE 54. Exercise for the abdominals.

6. Abdominals

Squeeze your abdominal region for 8 seconds, being careful to keep a flat stomach (don't push out) as you do it. Try to do this exercise several times a day.

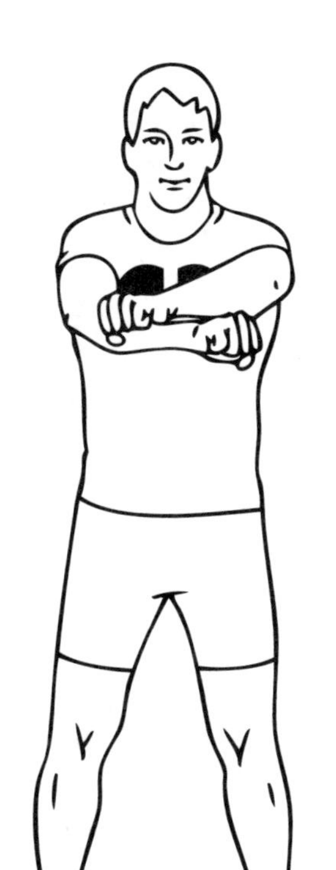

FIGURE 55. Exercise for the chest.

7. Chest

Cross one arm over the other as shown in the figure above. Squeeze your chest for 8 seconds.

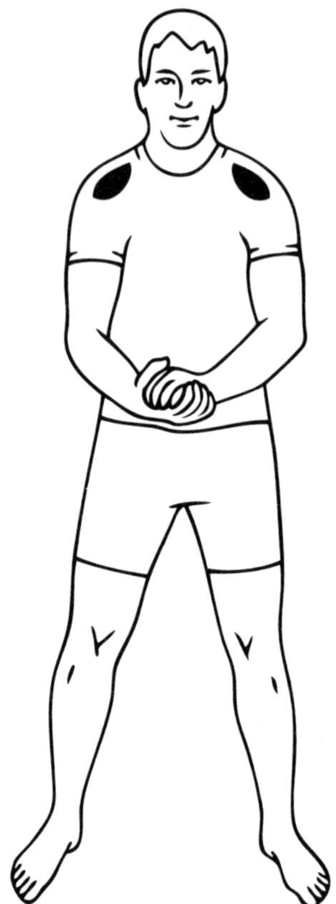

FIGURE 56. Exercise for the shoulders.

8. Shoulders

Slightly bend your arms and clasp one hand into the other, as if one hand is giving the other a handshake (see figure). If your right hand is on top, push it down, contracting and squeezing your right shoulder muscles. Hold for 4 seconds, then switch hand positions and switch to the other side, holding the contraction for 4 seconds. Repeat an additional set for each shoulder.

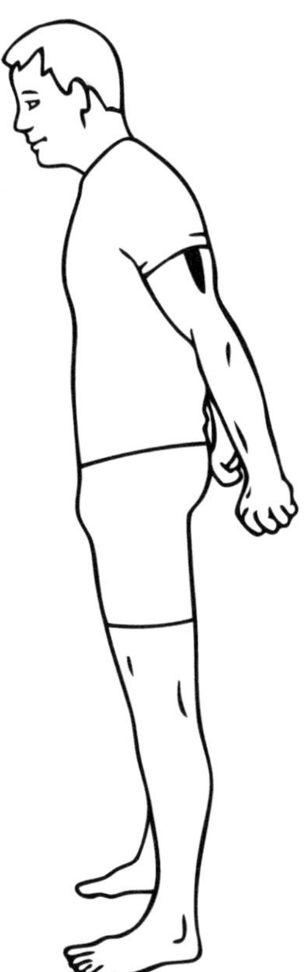

FIGURE 57. Exercise for the triceps.

9. Triceps

Your triceps are the muscles on the backs of your upper arms. Straighten both arms and hold them at a slight angle behind you as shown in the figure above. Now squeeze your entire arms tightly for 4 seconds. Release the contraction for 4 seconds, and then repeat the contraction for 4 more seconds.

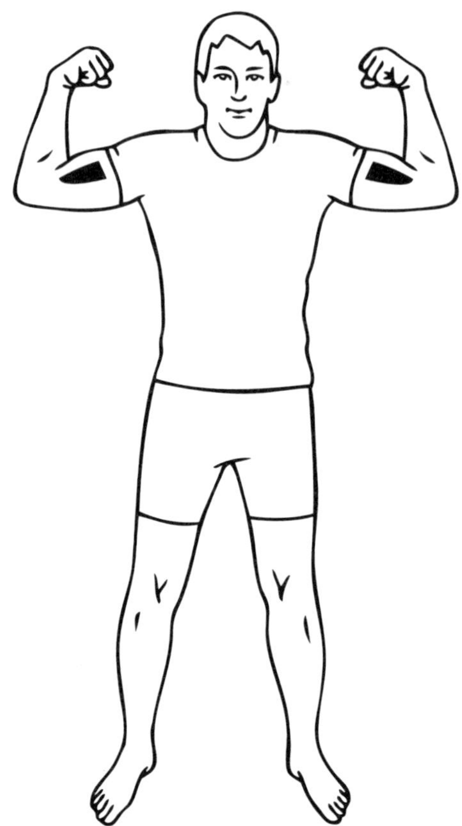

FIGURE 58. Exercise for the biceps.

10. Biceps

Biceps are the muscles on your inner upper arms. Lift both arms straight up until they're parallel with your shoulders, and then bend your arms in so your fists are now over your shoulders as shown in the figure above. Now contract and squeeze the biceps for 4 seconds, the way you would flex your biceps to show their size. Relax the contraction—let the arms straighten, still holding them at shoulder height. Then contract again for 4 seconds.

I believe in using your own body to perform all exercises, whether it be internal for your internal organs, or external, meaning musculoskeletal. (The only exception here is with the indispensable exercise of rebounding [see Chapter 16, The Miracle of Rebounding], because you do need equipment for that and you cannot mimic it otherwise.) Using your own body allows you to perform your exercise anywhere, any place, any time. I do mine in the shower in the morning—it is a great way to start the day. If you would like further guidance on isometric exercise or would like an isometrics exercise routine with energizing music, you may want to purchase my DVD, *The Isometric Total Body Workout.*™

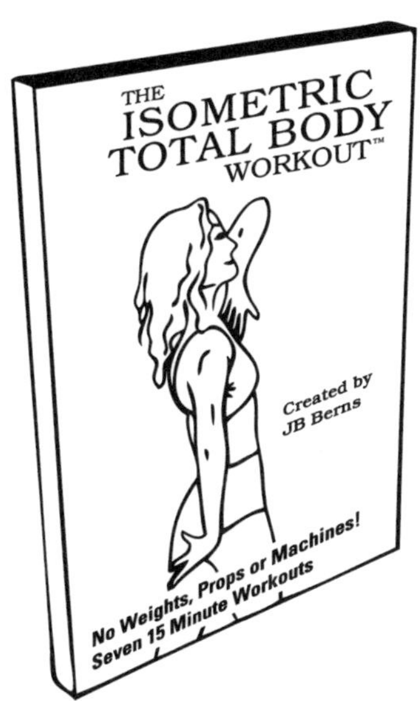

FIGURE 59. My DVD with additional isometric workouts to try.

The workouts in the video do not require weights, props, or fitness machines. All you will ever need to get in shape and stay in shape are these heart-pumping sculpting and toning workouts. You will finally look forward to exercise because it's easy and you will see quick, visible results, all in an environment of safe exercise protocol. There are no difficult postures, no jarring movements—and no pills or starvation diets, either.

Whether you do your exercises in the shower or in your exercise room with the DVD blaring, your routine need only take 60 seconds.

For more information on the DVD mentioned in this chapter, go to:
www.DOITORAGEQUICKLY.com
www.JBBERNS.com

7
HAIR HEALTH

For 60 Seconds:
Massage your scalp.

Our hair is a significant part of our appearance. It affects our self-confidence, our emotions, and our impressions upon other people. In this chapter I will address how to best enhance your hair through exercises, management, and products, as well as how to keep it as you age.

An excellent exercise for the scalp is included in Chapter 3, Internal Exercises. It's called the Hair Rubbing Exercise. The kneading pressure you will use with this massage will warm your skin and open your blood vessels to increase flow and boost circulation. Increased circulation means that the cells of the hair follicle will receive more of the nutrients necessary for optimal hair growth function, and it will keep your hair from falling out.

In the same vein, there is an excellent product on the market that takes this step even further. Buy the Marvy Shampoo Brush and Invigorator, a textured rubber disc you hold in the palm of your hand (see figure). Use it to massage your scalp for one minute a day. I usually use mine in the shower when washing my hair, but it doesn't matter, you can pick it up anytime and use it on dry hair as well. You can do the massage several times a day; do try to get it in at least once a day.

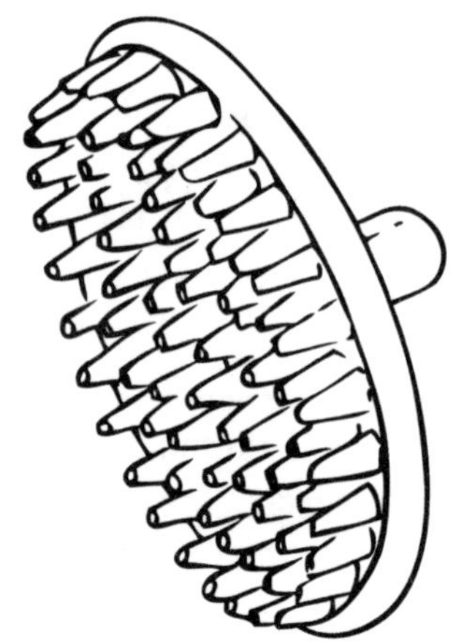

FIGURE 60. Shampoo brush and scalp invigorator.

When I do the massage with the brush I recommend, my scalp feels softer and my hair immediately appears thicker. I have been doing this for 20 years, and there is no doubt in my mind that it has slowed down the male pattern baldness that is in my lineage and DNA. It only costs about $6 and is well worth it! For purchasing information, see the websites listed at the end of this chapter.

The following herbal formula for the hair is called Royal Hair Ener-G, which is described (and created) by doctor and Taoist Stephen T. Chang in his book *The Great Tao*. It is to be used on your hair after you shower, when your pores are open.

It contains these ingredients:
Cypress, Elsha, Ginger, Sophora, Mint, Litzia

Here is a summary of what this formula can do for your hair and scalp:

- It restores health and balance to the scalp and hair cells with nutrients that specially benefit the hair.
- It naturally stimulates luxuriant hair growth.
- It gives hair shine, life, luster, and body.
- It soothes itchiness of the scalp and skin.

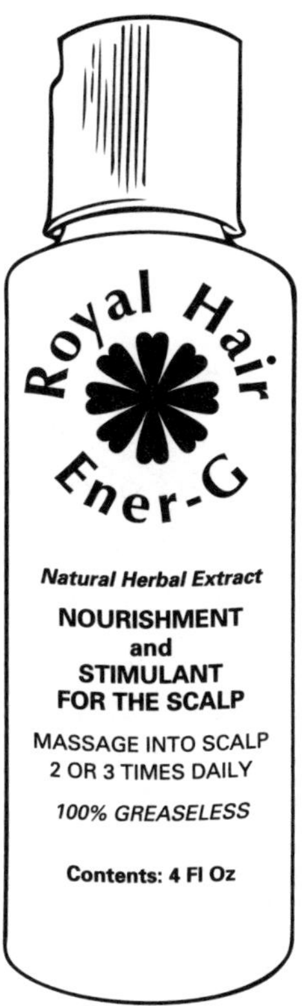

FIGURE 61. Royal Hair Energ-G natural herbal extract for the hair.

Royal Hair Ener-G is water soluble and gives the hair a natural shine without leaving a residue. It is not just for hair loss, so I highly recommend it for both men and women. It's for overall maintenance of the follicle, hair shaft, and scalp, and I strongly believe it is the best hair product on the market.

The reason I recommend Royal Hair Ener-G so highly is because my personal experience with it has been simply wonderful. I apply the liquid two times a day, usually after a warm shower so that the pores in my hair shaft are open. I then massage my scalp for 60 seconds. Over the many years of continual use, I have seen a reduction of hair loss and a strengthening of my hair follicles. In addition to conditioning the hair, Royal Hair Ener-G by Dr. Chang is an absolute must for all people who wish to slow down or stop their hair loss. See the end of this chapter for purchasing information.

Male Pattern Baldness

To focus on the men for a minute, I would like to discuss thinning hair, a topic most men over 30 are probably concerned about. For the majority of cases, male pattern baldness falls under the category of "androgenetic alopecia," which means that androgens are the underlying cause. Testosterone is an androgen and is responsible for sex characteristics in men, such as a deep voice and facial hair. When testosterone interacts with the enzyme 5-alpha reductase, it converts into dihydrotestosterone (DHT), a more potent version of testosterone. The problem is, hair follicles wither and die when exposed to DHT over time. Because of their genetics, some people have hair follicles that are very sensitive to DHT, which shortens the lifespan of the hair follicle.

Because of the DHT link, the first-line pharmaceutical treatment for male pattern baldness is 5-alpha reductase inhibitors (e.g., Propecia). Minoxidil (Rogaine), a blood vessel dilator, is considered the second most effective pharmaceutical treatment. However, diet, nutrition, and lifestyle have also been shown to affect hair loss as well as hair growth.

One of the most effective regimens I have found for the prevention of a receding hairline can be found in Dr. Cass Ingram's book *Eat Right or Die Young* (1989, Instant Improvement, Inc.). There are many claims out there, but most do not work. Following this system may stop the hair loss associated with male pattern baldness and, in some cases, may stimulate new hair growth.

1. **Control stress.** Worrying and stress cause the muscles in the scalp to tighten, which cuts off blood flow in the hair follicles. Please read Chapter 2, Ten Deep Breaths, for excellent, natural techniques in reducing tension and stress.
2. **Use a shampoo containing pure herbal extracts.** I believe the best is Shampure by Aveda. Shampure is flower- and plant-based and gentle. It also contains sources of essential fatty acids (such as avocado oil), which are valuable for promoting strong, healthy hair shafts. It costs about $10.
3. **Wash hair with cold water.** If you wash your hair with warm water the pores become open and the hair shaft can slip out. Cold water will also create a better shine for the hair.
4. **Take Tuna Omega-3 Oil (by Standard Process).** There is some evidence that saturated fat exacerbates hair loss in men. Tuna Omega-3 Oil will help counter this by adding healthy fats to your system. Cutting down on the red meat couldn't hurt, either! (See the end of this chapter for purchasing information.)

Care for your hair—it's so easy and takes only 60 seconds.

For more information on hair care, go to:
www.DOITORAGEQUICKLY.com
www.JBBERNS.com

8

FACIAL PRODUCTS TO PRESERVE AND HEAL

For 60 Seconds:
Exfoliate your face with Royal Vital Clean-Off, and then use the Royal S.A.R. Gold, Royal Essence of Pearl, and Royal Jade lotions.

The following are four facial products prescribed by Dr. Stephen T. Chang in *The Great Tao* that I highly recommend. They do wonders for skin tone and texture and comprehensively work on all of the things we'd rather not have on our face, like dry skin, wrinkles, and blemishes.

I have tried them all, and trust me, you cannot buy better facial products to slow down the aging process of your face than the products I will describe in this chapter: Royal Vital Clean-Off, a gentle, everyday exfoliator, Royal S.A.R. Gold Lotion, Royal Essence of Pearl, and Royal Jade Cream. Nothing comes close. They are all a must to keep in your medicine cabinet and your pocketbook or pocket (to be applied several times throughout the day). The products make skin look younger, more toned, richer in color, and more soft and supple. If you cut your skin shaving or develop a pimple, this facial care system will speed up the recovery and healing time. I have been using them for 20 years and cannot endorse them enough.

These products can be used at any time, but if you only do the routine once a day, they are especially effective if incorporated into your nighttime routine. First cleanse your face with Vital Clean-Off, then wring out a hot washcloth and lay it on your face for a few minutes to open your pores. Let your skin dry for a minute, and then apply S.A.R. Gold Lotion with one finger to potential wrinkle areas such as your eyes and forehead. Next, apply a thin layer of Essence of Pearl, and let it dry. Finally, follow with Jade Cream, covering your whole face.

Note that you should apply a greater amount of Jade Cream to certain acupressure points. Gently massage the areas around your eyes by lightly moving your fingertips in a circle around your eyes 36 times, starting from the eyebrows and moving outward. Next, rub your palms together to generate heat, and then place them on your eyes. This procedure prevents the formation of wrinkles and gives the skin a natural glow. The cream also preserves the youth of the skin cells.

You can apply these products throughout the day, up to two to three times total. I recommend that you do the entire procedure twice a day, once in the morning when you awake and again before you go to bed at night. For men and women who don't wear makeup, apply during the day as well to maximize the benefits.

Below are the products I recommend with their ingredients and benefits.

- Royal Vital Clean-Off
- Royal S.A.R. Gold Lotion
- Royal Essence of Pearl
- Royal Jade Cream

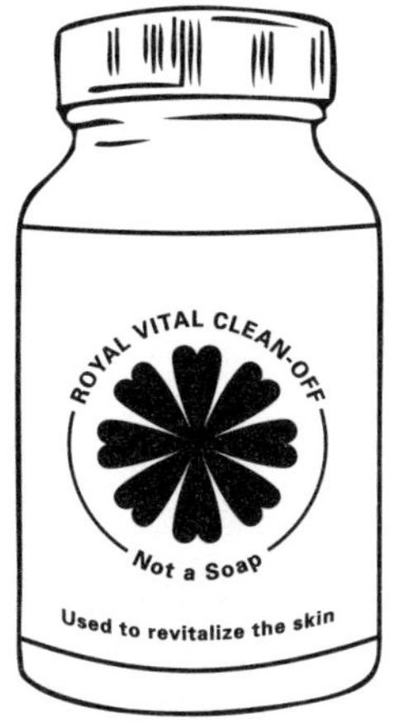

FIGURE 62. Vital Clean-Off

Royal Vital Clean-Off

Vital Clean-Off is a superb exfoliator that sloughs off dead tissue and deeply cleanses the skin and pores. It is made up of natural, healing herbs that penetrate, soften, and revitalize the skin. It also functions to protect and heal the skin, which makes shaving easier and less abrasive.

The formula contains these active ingredients:
Nepeta, Kuta, Sophora, Alumen, Milk

It is a powder that contains no preservatives or chemicals, which forms a substrate hostile to the growth of microorganisms.

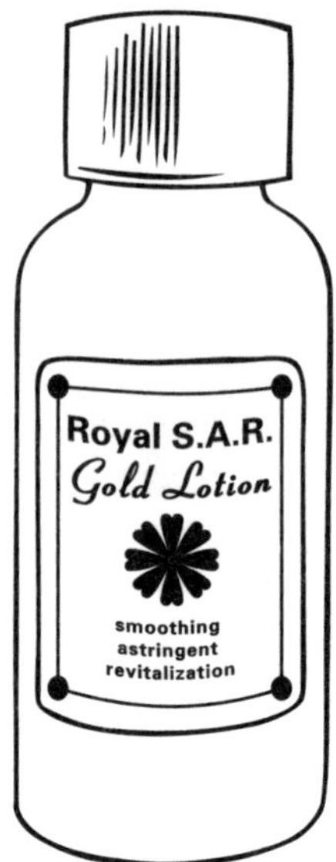

FIGURE 63. S.A.R. Gold Lotion

Royal S.A.R. Gold Lotion

S.A.R. stands for Skin Astringent and Repair. This combination contains these treasured ingredients:
Liquid Gold, Royal Jelly, Asparagus (herb), Ginseng

- It smoothes and refines the texture of the skin.
- It prevents the formation of wrinkles.
- It controls oiliness and dryness with special corrective, balancing ingredients.
- It revitalizes tired skin and gives it life and health.
- It's antiseptic.

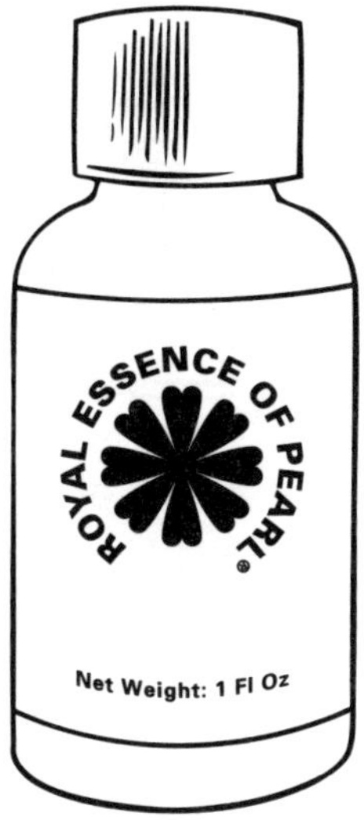

FIGURE 64. Essence of Pearl facial conditioner.

Royal Essence of Pearl

Pearls have been known for centuries in Asia for their skin beautifying properties. This facial conditioner contains natural moisturizers that are immediately absorbed by the skin because of their similarity to natural skin fluids.

Essence of Pearl contains these ingredients:
Pearls, Ginseng, Ginkgo, Almond seed extract, Cotylegon

- Essence of Pearl beautifies skin conditions with its combination of herbal conditioners.
- It makes the skin unbelievably soft, radiant, and youthful.
- Its unique ingredient qualities increase vitality to the skin.

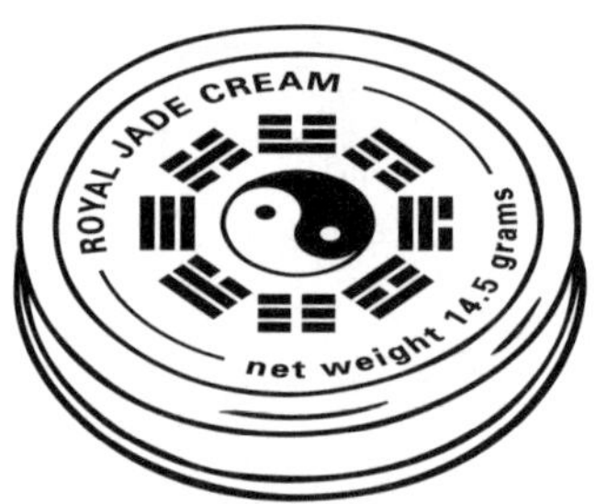

FIGURE 65. Jade Cream.

Royal Jade Cream

In the spirit of Taoist principles, an extraordinary herbal skin care system was developed for the royal families of China centuries ago. The herbal combinations they were made of were so treasured that they were more precious than priceless gems. This particular combination has been famous in the history of China.

Jade Cream contains these exquisite materials:
Jade, Lithospermum, Frankincense, Myrrh, Pearls, Sesame oil

It heals and regenerates new cells and tissue and can be used to treat blemishes, scars, wrinkles, and damaged skin. It can be used on any skin area—face or body, day or night, and only a small amount is needed.

- Jade Cream helps generate new, healthy skin tissue and repairs old, unhealthy cells.
- It helps removes scars, wrinkles, and blemishes.
- It makes the skin healthy and look radiant.
- The physicians of the Royal Family of China have also reported a wide range of benefits from Royal Jade Cream for symptoms like (or resembling): joints deformed by arthritis, herpes, sprained ankles, psoriasis, breast lumps,

vaginal infections, skin cancer, spinal dysfunction, hemorrhoids, cataracts, glaucoma, and eczema. Its effectiveness has been continuously proven over the centuries.

- It can also be used internally for gum infections, canker sores, hemorrhoids, herpes, and some eye diseases.
- It forms a protective barrier from the effects of the wind, cold, and pollution.
- Jade Cream is a superior product for treating infant diaper rash and skin irritations.

Note that people with oily skin should not use Royal Jade Cream. If you have oily skin, use only Essence of Pearl in the beginning to remedy it. When your skin is no longer oily, proceed with Jade Cream after Essence of Pearl.

Use the products mentioned here and watch your facial skin improve like you have never seen it before.

For more information on the products mentioned in this chapter, go to:
www.DOITORAGEQUICKLY.com
www.JBBERNS.com

9

THE HERBAL FOUNTAIN OF YOUTH

For 60 Seconds:
Drink these herbal formulas for energy and youth.

Western medicine tends to focus on diagnosing a disorder and then treating it. On the other hand, Eastern medicine, Taoists in particular, are focused on keeping the body in balance and strengthening the entire body. Because balance is such an integral concept, over the centuries Taoist research has discarded any method with side effects, as the correction of one function at the expense of another does not re-establish balance. The goal is to strengthen the physical, mental, and spiritual parts of an individual, all at the same time.

The herbal formulas listed below (one combination for women and one for men) have been created with the above in mind and benefit many different systems of the body. They are essentially a fountain of youth and will change your life. They will slow down the aging process by keeping your body balanced and filled with the rare nutrients that are in these unique formulas. The listed commentaries represent symptoms or diseases associated with a certain abnormal state of the body's function. Both herbal combinations have been associated with a series of symptoms that according to Western science would be unrelated. However, the Taoist emphasis is on promoting the body's ability to repair itself and prevent or correct an abnormal state rather than focusing on symptoms and diseases.

I can't comment on the women's reproductive formula from first-hand experience, but the women I know who are taking this formula state that it is the most important thing they consume each day, and they swear by its fountain of youth results with zero side effects. I can personally say that the regeneration tea for men is simply a godsend. I take it two to three times a day—one teaspoon of the powder followed by a glass of water on an empty stomach (or you can mix it with hot water). It has given me greater natural energy coupled with a healthy sexual drive. It's very important for all men and women to take and a necessity in the system of this book. Each bottle is roughly $50, but it will be the best money you ever spend. I've been taking regeneration tea for over 20 years, and I am sincere when I say it is the fountain of youth. Both formulas balance your body internally. Many women report that they experience a strong sexual drive and energy, comparable to what men experience. A side note: Don't be intimidated by the taste of the powder; make a tea of it, and train your body and mind to like the taste.

One of the reasons it's so important for men and women to take their respective formulas of healing herbs is that you cannot find them in ordinary foods. Many are ingredients passed on from ancient times. These Chinese formulas can be found in the old pharmaceutical books. An herbalist could re-create them, but he or she would need to find and purchase all of the herbs and rare ingredients. This is why I buy Dr. Chang's premade organic powders from his Tao Healing Arts company. They are made in Asia and distributed by his company in the United States. For more information on how to purchase them, please see the end of this chapter.

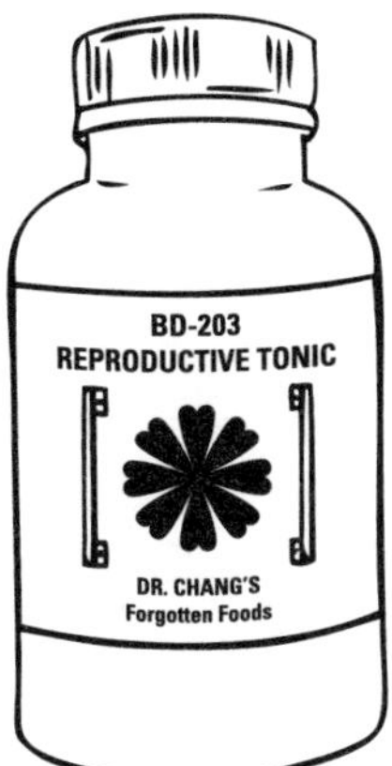

FIGURE 66. Reproductive tonic for women.

Female Formula: BD-203, Reproductive Tonic Combination

This strengthens and balances the female reproductive organs and hormonal system. Its benefits are far-reaching and connected to the body as a whole.

- **Ingredients:** Tang Kuei, Cnidium, Paeonia, Poria, Atractylodes, Alisma, Sargentia
- **Combination's Energy Level:** Neutral
- **Combination's Taste:** 45% sweet (affects spleen-pancreas), 15% piquant (affects lungs), 15% sour (affects liver), 15% bitter (affects heart), 10% salty (affects kidney)
- **Main Meridians:** Heart and spleen-pancreas

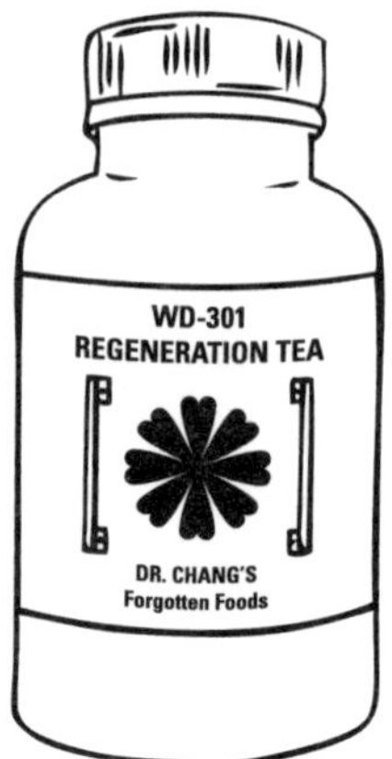

FIGURE 67. Regeneration tea for men.

Male Formula: WD-301, Regeneration Combination

This herbal combination is best taken as a tea or directly in powder form in your mouth (followed with a drink of water). It is especially potent in boosting immunity, which affects day-to-day health as well as long-term health and lifespan. Its benefits are broad, balancing the male body as a whole.

- **Ingredients:** Rhemannia, Cornia, Doiscorea, Alisma, Poria, Suffructicosa, Cinnamon, Aconite
- **Combination's Energy Level:** Neutral
- **Combination's Taste:** 65% sweet (affects spleen-pancreas), 30% salty (affects kidney), 5% piquant (affects lungs)
- **Main Meridians:** Rather balanced, but primarily sedates heart and also liver; energizes stomach, lungs, and kidneys

Through modern technology we have the gift of having these incredible formulas organically bottled for our consumption. Please take advantage of this wonderful gift.

Note: *If you have any concerns, it is advisable to consult your physician before using these herbal combinations.*

To purchase either of the herbal formulas spoken of in this chapter, go to:
www.DOITORAGEQUICKLY.com
www.JBBERNS.com

10

THE BEST VITAMINS MONEY CAN BUY

For 60 Seconds:
Take your vitamins: Tuna Omega-3 Oil, Andrographis Complex, bilberry, ginkgo biloba, garlic, and hawthorn.

Most of you know what a healthy diet entails: lots of fruits and vegetables, whole grains, legumes, nuts and seeds, healthy fats, a little dairy, and a little lean fish or meat. What makes this so healthy? Can you distill the essence of these elements into a pill? The answers to these questions are, respectively, we don't completely know, and not likely.

Scientists have carefully studied the foods and their components of the healthiest, longest living people in the world. While there are many theories that likely explain it, we still don't have all of the answers, because we still aren't able to bottle it. In other words, it is something about eating the whole foods and the components of the diet in tandem that delivers the most benefits. Most vitamin supplement studies show that supplements do not offer nearly the benefits that a healthy diet as described above does. (Note that we are not talking about undernourished subjects taking a vitamin they are known to be deficient in.)

Take phytochemicals as an example. Phytochemicals are non-nutrient plant chemicals that give fruits and vegetables their different tastes and colors. They are also antioxidants and have been associated with the reduction of chronic diseases such as high blood pressure, diabetes, Alzheimer's, heart disease, and cancer, among other maladies. A diet rich in fruits and vegetables provides hundreds of phytochemicals, possibly even 25,000 or more. Because we haven't even begun to identify all of them yet, we can't possibly replicate all of what makes them healthy in a pill, either.

The next best option to obtaining all of the healthy nutrients available from foods is to supplement with whole-food vitamins. As the name implies, these are vitamins made by concentrating whole foods for use in supplements. When processed correctly, they supply a multitude of the plant's components. Since most of us don't eat nearly as healthy a diet as we should, whole-food supplements supply our bodies with the nutrients we are not getting—the vitamins, minerals, trace minerals, and phytochemicals, in all of their complexity.

Since you cannot take hundreds of pills a day, I don't advise striving for comprehensive coverage. Rather, there are a handful that are best for a normal, healthy person (if you have any health conditions you should discuss these supplements with your physician before taking them).

I recommend the following mixture of supplements for everyday consumption.

- Tuna Omega-3 Oil
- Andrographis Complex
- Bilberry
- Ginkgo Biloba
- Garlic
- Hawthorn

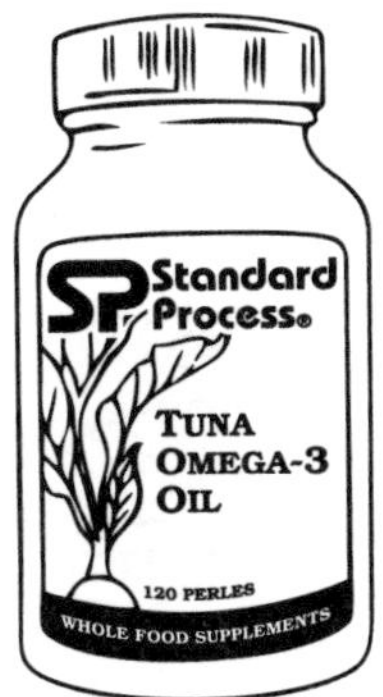

FIGURE 68.
Tuna Omega-3 Oil by Standard Process.

Tuna Omega-3 Oil for the Heart

Omega-3 fatty acids are very beneficial to your health, yet most Americans do not ingest nearly enough of them. They are implicated in helping prevent cardiovascular disease and cancer, and they may help improve inflammatory conditions such as arthritis as well as many mental conditions.

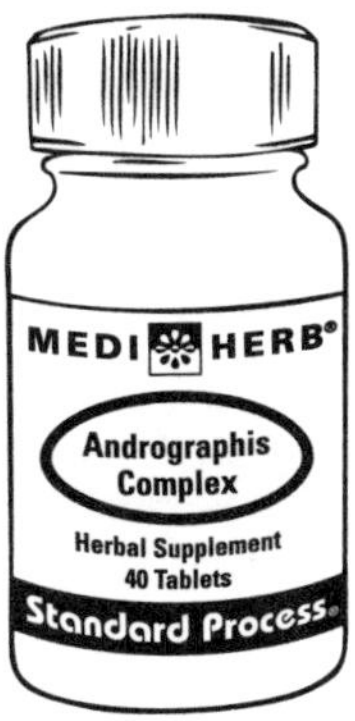

FIGURE 69.
Andrographis Complex.

Andrographis Complex for the Immune System

This herbal combination (which includes Echinacea and is made by MediHerb) is designed to support and enhance many aspects of the immune system; it may be particularly beneficial in treating upper respiratory infections. (*It is contraindicated in pregnancy and lactation as well as allergy to plants of the daisy family.*)

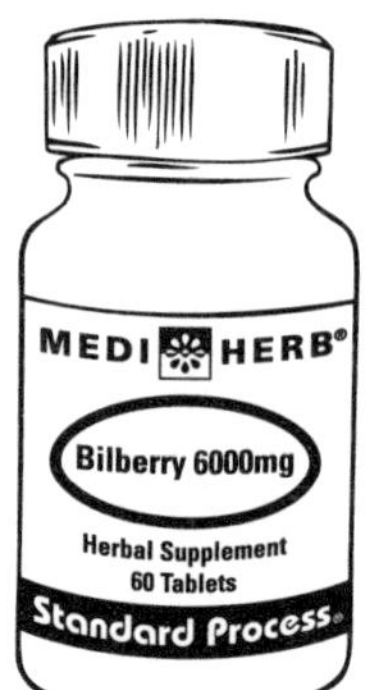

FIGURE 70.
Bilberry tablets.

Bilberry for the Eyes

In addition to helping maintain healthy eyes, this byproduct of bilberries appears to help the circulatory system as well. (See more about this in Chapter 11, Eye Health.)

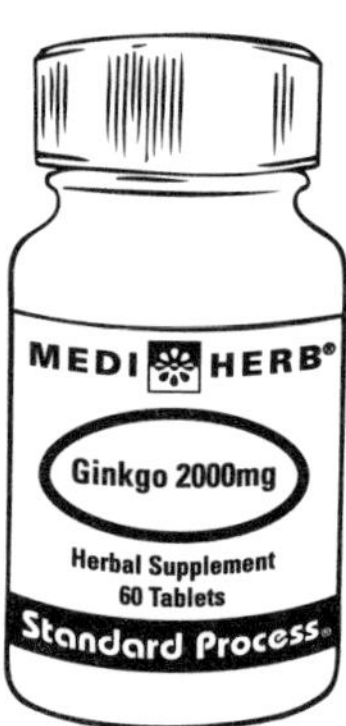

FIGURE 71.
Ginkgo biloba tablets.

Ginkgo Biloba for Memory

Extracts from the ginkgo biloba plant are thought to stimulate healthy brain function through increased circulation and oxygenation; it appears to enhance attention and memory, and it may generally help the circulatory system. (*Caution: This product is not to be used by pregnant or lactating women.*)

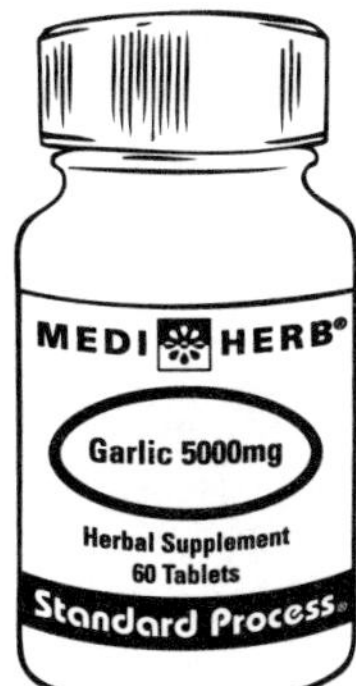

FIGURE 72.
Garlic tablets.

Garlic Tablets for Detoxifying

Garlic is a powerful antioxidant and protector against damage from free radicals, which are molecules that injure cells and may be responsible for inappropriate cell division and growth; thus garlic may improve the cardiovascular and immune systems in particular and aid in preventing cancer. (Note that the beneficial phytochemicals in garlic may degrade after cooking.)

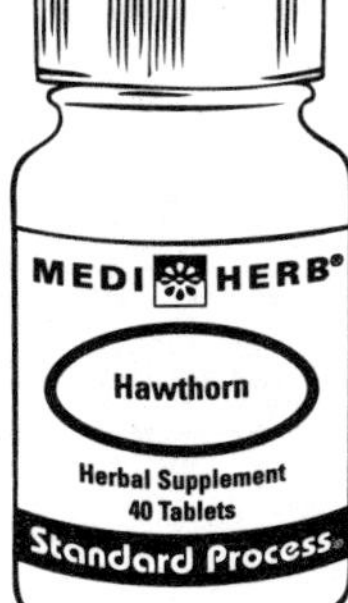

FIGURE 73.
Hawthorn tablets.

Hawthorn for the Heart

Hawthorn supports the functioning of healthy heart muscle; scientific evidence shows that it is beneficial in cases of mild heart failure.

I strongly believe that Standard Process is far and away the best company from which to purchase supplements, and it is where all of the above supplements can be found. Standard Process has been around since 1929 and has a Research & Development department of scientists who work to provide a solid scientific basis for the supplements they carry. They utilize the best growing practices available and use nothing but the finest, high-quality organic food supplements and vitamins.

All of the supplements described above are Standard Process products or a MediHerb product, which is exclusively distributed through Standard Process and has an advanced Research & Development department of its own. All of the vitamins described above are sometimes difficult to find in health stores due to their high distribution standards, so I am making them available for purchase through my website (see below).

Increase your energy, health, and lifespan: Take your Standard Process vitamins as part of your morning routine so you won't forget.

For more information on the vitamins mentioned in this chapter, go to:
www.DOITORAGEQUICKLY.com
www.JBBERNS.com

11

EYE HEALTH

For 60 Seconds:
Massage your eyes, study an eye chart, and supplement with bilberry tablets.

An eye doctor I know once commented that whenever a patient is having eye trouble, he or she will say, "Doc, I gotta be able to see better, my eyes are so important to my work!" The truth is that it doesn't matter if you work as a librarian, at a manufacturing plant, as a stay-at-home mom, or as a neurosurgeon, we *all* are incredibly dependent upon our vision.

Many people have had faulty vision since they were children. And most people will notice deterioration as they age—the print seems to get smaller and smaller, until the time comes to buy some reading glasses or bifocals. I believe, however, that this deleterious path is avoidable. Your eyes do not have to follow this course, and you may even be able to improve the faulty vision you have been accustomed to, if you follow my recommendations and regularly perform the eye exercises I describe in this chapter.

About 20 years ago I began to feel my vision weaken ever so slightly. As a result, I did a little research and asked my teacher and mentor Dr. Stephen Chang (an M.D.) what he recommended to slow down the deterioration of my vision and the overall aging of my eyes. What I learned, which has essentially stabilized my vision, was a palm-rubbing eye-soothing technique, and about six acupressure points in my eyes that I can massage with my fingertips.

I began massaging my eyes using these methods each and every day for 60 seconds, followed by the palming technique. I perform these exercises as part of my internal exercise routine every morning; you can find descriptions of them in Chapter 3, Internal Exercises. Within about one week of starting the acupressure massage and palming my eyes, I began to feel my vision strengthen and my focus become much clearer. My eyes felt as if they had more energy every time I did the acupressure massage and palming. The exercises can also help cosmetically, reducing bags or puffiness under the eyes.

In addition to the above exercises, you can also enhance your eye health by reading a standard eye chart once a day for 60 seconds. Stand about 15 feet away from it and read with one eye while the other is closed, and vice versa. This is primarily for the maintenance of your vision and may help improve it as well.

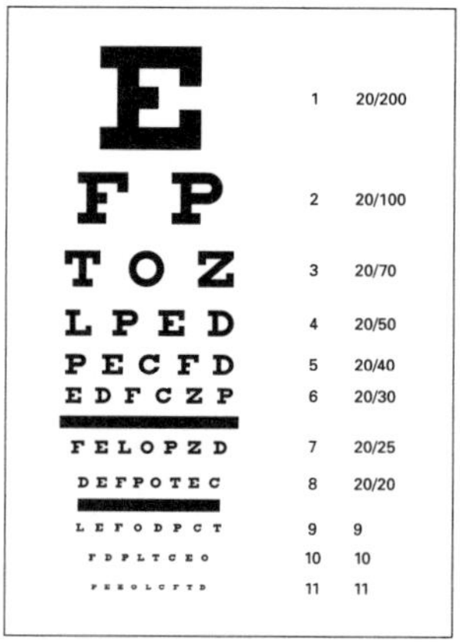

FIGURE 74. Eye chart for eye strengthening exercises.

I would also like to call your attention to the natural eye drops product, Similasan Dry Eye Relief eye drops, pictured below. This is a wonderful product that can be used at any age to lubricate and moisturize your eyes. Vasoconstrictors are often an ingredient in over-the-counter eye drops (such as Visine and Murine) to treat red eyes; they work by causing the blood vessels to shrink. Doctors do not recommend prolonged usage of these products, however, as it can lead to dryness of the eyes, increased swelling, rebound redness, and conjunctivitis. By contrast, Similasan eye drops do not contain vasoconstrictors nor other harsh chemicals, and therefore do not cause such side effects. They work naturally, stimulating the eye's natural ability to fight dryness and irritation and to clear redness due to smog, stress, age, contact lenses, and so on.

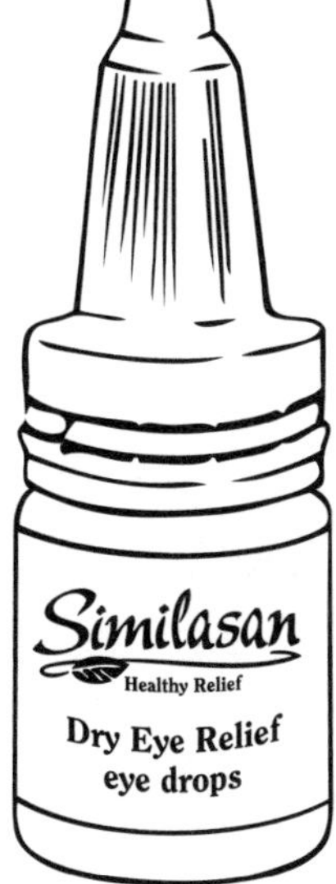

FIGURE 75. Similasan eye drops.

My final recommendation to support your vision is to take Standard Process bilberry tablets (see Chapter 10, The Best Vitamins Money Can Buy, to learn more about Standard Process supplements and where to get them). Part of the evidence supporting its benefit to the eyes is found in its help in preventing the onset and progress of two age-related eye diseases that can greatly impair vision: cataracts and macular degeneration. Cataracts are a clouding of the lens, and macular degeneration causes a gradual loss of vision in the center of one's focal field. They both affect a very large number of people and can be a devastating development for the sufferer. However, studies suggest that natural remedies can help.

Both cataracts and macular degeneration have been shown to be related to oxidative stress. Thus, antioxidant therapy has been suggested as a method to prevent or slow their development. In fact, studies show that a diet rich in fruits and vegetables (naturally high in antioxidants) do have this effect.

The fruit bilberries are thought to be particularly effective. Bilberries are related to blueberries, which have one of the highest antioxidant content of all fruits and vegetables. Bilberries neutralize free radical damage to the collagen matrix of cells and tissues that can lead to cataracts and glaucoma, and they may help protect against macular degeneration as well. Both fruits are deep blue in color due to dense levels of anthocyanin pigments. Anthocyanins are known to be powerful antioxidants, which may be where the protective effect of bilberries comes from. Preliminary studies in rats have shown that bilberry extract can have a profound effect in preventing both cataracts and macular degeneration.

So what if you don't have fresh bilberries available in your area? What about bilberry supplements? While some studies of antioxidant supplements suggest that they do not help prevent eye diseases, others show that they may slow down the process once a person has one. It should be noted that these supplements (such as vitamin E or beta-carotene) were isolated, artificially made supplements. The difference with Standard Process supplements (which I highly recommend), such as those for bilberry, contain whole-food concentrate. Thus, when you take Standard Process bilberry supplements, you are receiving the whole benefit of the fruit, so the effects would likely imitate the whole fruit and extract studies.

As I say, I have been following the above regimen for 20 years. I am now 40-plus and still do not wear glasses. I sincerely believe it is due to my eye maintenance, because my whole family has poor eyesight and wears glasses, along with my father, who has macular degeneration. I only wish I had stressed my gold nuggets of eye health to family members 20 years ago! What I can do is say to them now, and to you: Better late than never!

For more information on the products mentioned in this chapter, go to:
www.DOITORAGEQUICKLY.com
www.JBBERNS.com

12
EIGHT ENERGIZING EXERCISES

For 60 Seconds:
Perform the eight directional exercises facing northwest, north, northeast, east, southeast, south, southwest, and west.

The Taoists find continuity between the physical inanimate world and mankind. And why shouldn't they? Everything is governed by the same rules of physics, and is composed of atoms from the same periodic table, which at their most fundamental are built from energy. One of the rules of physics is that where there is mass, there is direction. And where there are electric forces, there is direction. After much experimentation, the Taoists designed the following exercises for human beings to recharge and attain maximum energy, which include very specific instructions for the direction in which you perform the exercise. For this reason Taoists refer to them as "directional exercises."

When your body is energized, you don't feel tired, matters of the mind become simplified, you're able to solve business problems much more easily, and your body's durability increases. My Taoist mentor Dr. Stephen Chang advised me to add these exercises to my routine, which I did many years ago. I feel very strongly that these directional exercises should be included in your daily routine as well. The series of movements clears my mind and makes my body feel wonderful. In addition, I find the postures fun to perform and easy to do. Carefully determine which direction is north, preferably with a compass, before you begin.

I feel the best time to perform the eight directional exercises is early in the morning, right after a warm shower and/or anytime you feel tired during the day and want an extra burst of energy. I perform about seven repetitions of each exercise, although you can do as many or as little as you wish; there is no magic number of repetitions for the exercise series to be effective. Each exercise can be modified if you cannot mimic the exact movement in the drawing. For example, touching your hands to the floor is not completely necessary. One option would be to bend your legs and reach your hands down as close to the floor as you can get.

Below is my list of directional exercises that you should perform every day (instructions and diagrams to follow).

1. Northwest
2. North
3. Northeast
4. East
5. Southeast
6. South
7. Southwest
8. West

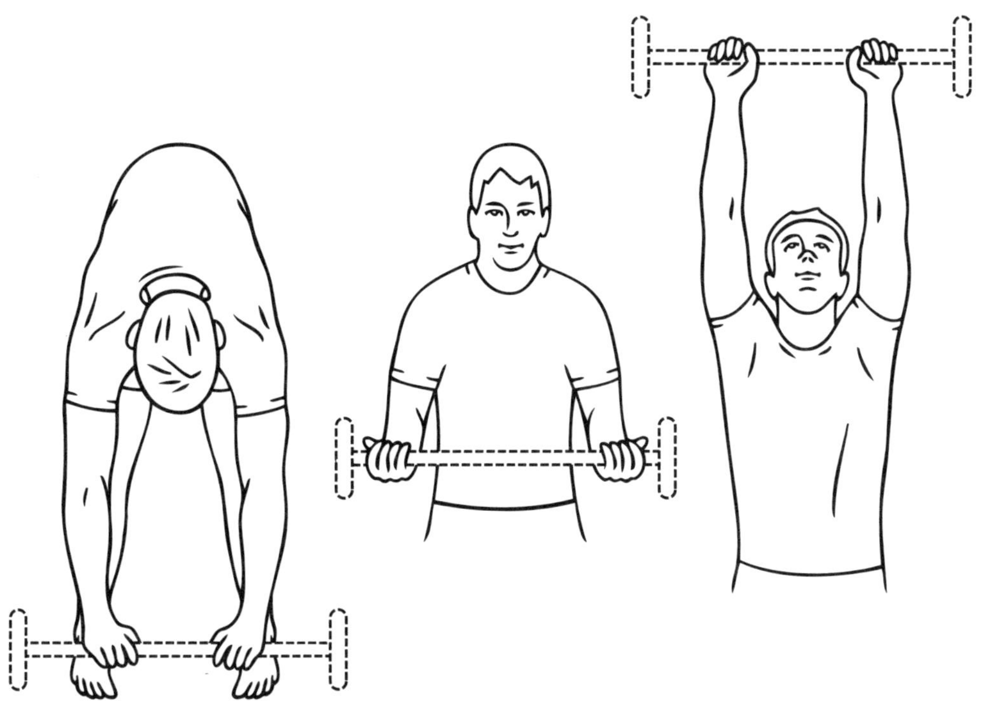

FIGURE 76. The northwestern exercise.

1. Northwest

For the northwestern directional exercise, face northwest. Stand with your feet shoulder-width apart, standing evenly on both feet with your toes pointed inward. Now, keeping your back and legs straight, bend over and lean down as if you're clasping an imaginary barbell. Clearly visualize this and focus on what you are doing. As if it were of medium weight (don't overstrain yourself), "lift" the barbell to waist level, and then "lift" it high overhead as far as it will go. Now do the exercise again but in reverse, starting from the top and repeating the movement in the opposite direction. Repeat as many times as you wish. This exercise should increase your strength and help your lungs and large intestines.

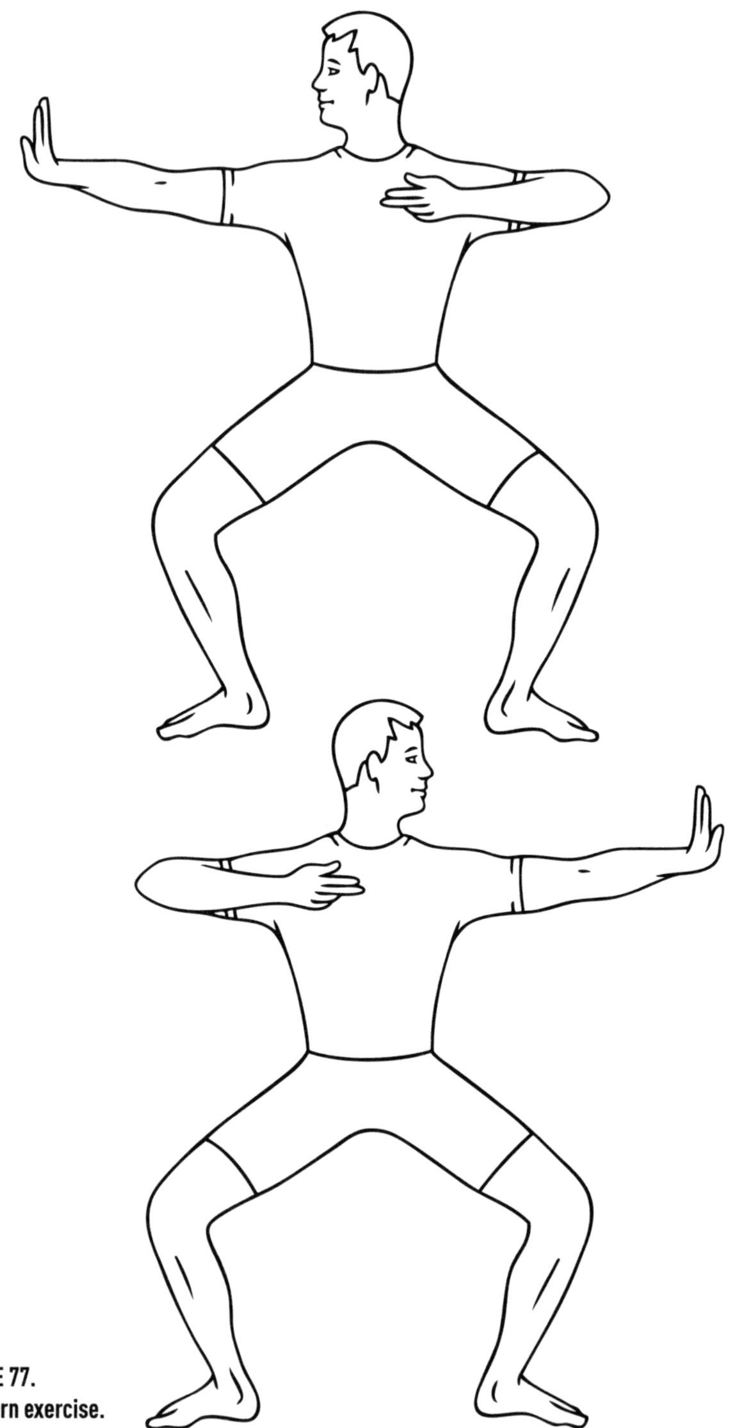

FIGURE 77.
Northern exercise.

2. North

For the northern exercise, face north. Keeping your torso facing north, spread your feet wide apart and pretend you are shooting an arrow from a bow to the side, as in Figure 77. Focus and clearly visualize that you are pulling on a taut bow and shooting the arrow. Now switch sides and shoot the arrow in the other direction (e.g., left versus right), keeping your feet and lower body stationary. Do the exercise as many times as you like. This exercise benefits your lungs, kidneys, large intestine, bladder, skin, and bones.

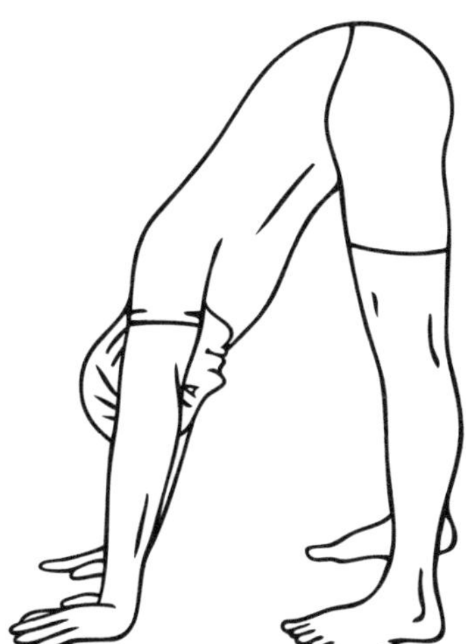

FIGURE 78.
Northeastern exercise.

3. Northeast

For the northeast directional exercise, stand facing in the northeastern direction with your legs shoulder-width apart. Keeping your back and legs straight, bend at your waist as much as you can and try to touch your toes with your fingertips. If you can bend even further, stretch in front of you as shown in the figure above and flatten your palms to the floor. Visualize that you are a mountain and hold this position for as long as you like. This exercise benefits the spleen, pancreas, and overall digestion.

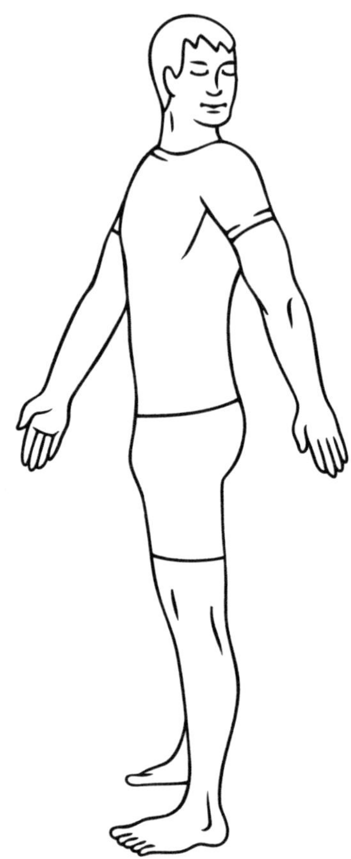

FIGURE 79.
Eastern exercise.

4. East

For the eastern directional exercise, if possible, do it in the morning under the sunlight, facing east, of course. Stand with your feet shoulder-width apart, toes pointed inward, and eyes closed. Keeping your feet and lower body stationary, let your hands fall to your sides, and turn your entire upper body to one side as shown in the figure above. Let your head turn with your torso. While your eyes are closed, let your eyeballs trace the source of radiant heat emitted by the sun as your head turns. Focus on what you're doing and don't let your mind wander. Do the exercise as long as you like. This exercise benefits the nerves, liver, eyes, and gallbladder, and aids in weight reduction.

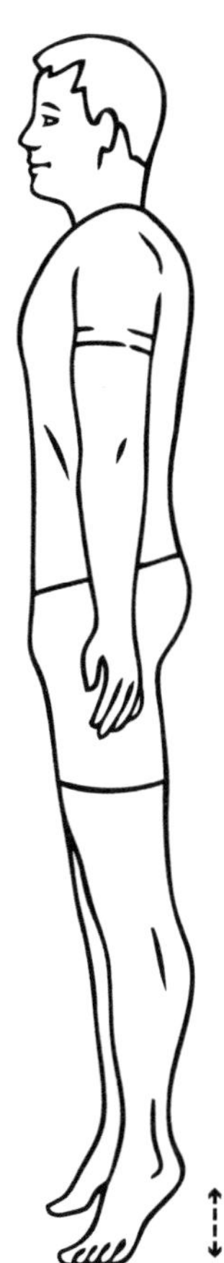

FIGURE 80.
Southeastern exercise.

5. Southeast

For the southeastern directional exercise, face your body southeast. Stand with your feet shoulder-width apart with your toes pointed inward. Lift yourself onto your toes, then lower yourself. Do seven complete sets. As in all of these exercises, focus on what you're doing while you're doing it and repeat as many times as you like. This exercise benefits the nerves, liver, gallbladder, and heart.

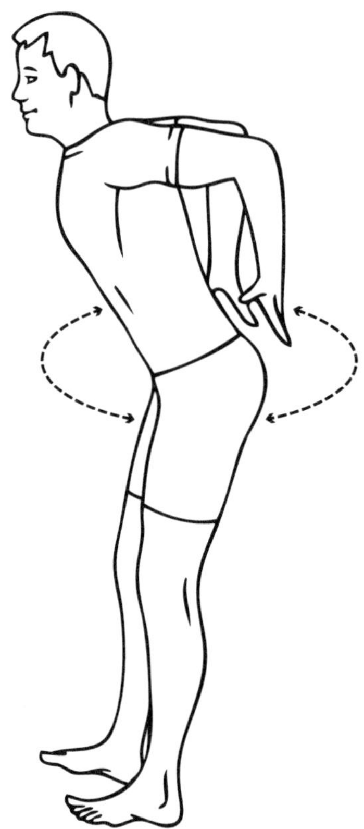

FIGURE 81. Southern exercise.

6. South

For the southern directional exercise, face your body directly south. Stand with your feet shoulder-width apart and rotate your hips in a circle as if you were twirling a hula-hoop around your hips. You may change the direction in which you rotate and continue as long as you wish. Focus on what you are doing and don't let your mind wander. This exercise benefits the sexual organs.

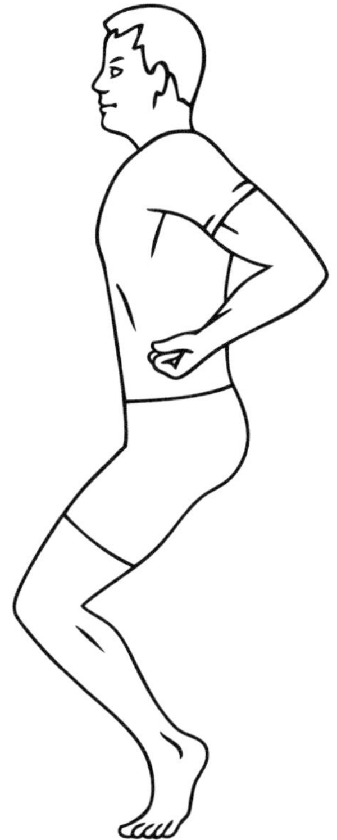

FIGURE 82. Southwestern exercise.

7. Southwest

For the southwestern directional exercise, face southwest. Bend at your knees slightly, bend your arms slightly, and clench your fists. Now rise up on your toes and imagine you are about to fight someone. Bulge your eyes out with rage. Focus on what you are doing; your mind must be with your body. Hold the pose as long as you like. This exercise is good for the digestive system, lungs, and nerves.

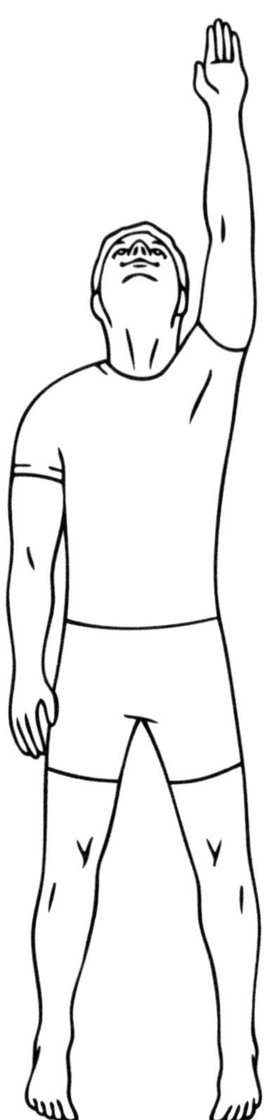

FIGURE 83.
Western exercise.

8. West

For the western directional exercise, face west. Stand with your legs shoulder-width apart and your toes pointed slightly inward. Raise one hand high in the air, keeping your arm straight. Now bring this hand down and raise your other hand. As you do this, try to keep your torso and abdomen still, and focus closely on what you are doing. Repeat as many times as you like. This exercise helps ease lower back pain, shoulder pain, kidney problems, and spinal problems.

Energize your tired mind and body with these eight simple exercises, it just takes 60 seconds.

For more information on the directional exercises mentioned in this chapter, go to:
www.DOITORAGEQUICKLY.com
www.JBBERNS.com

13

THREE ANIMAL EXERCISES

For 60 Seconds:
Perform your Animal Exercises—the crane, turtle, and deer exercises.

I refer to this chapter's recommended exercises collectively as the "Animal Exercises:" in the Taoist tradition they are called the Crane, Turtle, and Deer Exercises and work together to bring harmony to your physical body, mental body, and spiritual body. Thousands of years ago Taoist sages studied and emulated these three animals for their strength and longevity. To break it down, the Crane Exercises will strengthen and stimulate your circulatory and digestive systems. If these two systems are strong, then your body will be strong, you will feel strong, and your body will better resist illness and disease. The Turtle Exercises energize the nerves and strengthen the brain, spinal column, and neck region. Possessing a strong central nervous system will help you balance your mental energy, and over time it can help bring peace of mind. The Deer Exercises stimulate your physical and spiritual being. They will improve your sexual energy and support a balanced glandular and hormonal system for both men and women (there are different exercises for each).

My first experience doing the three Animal Exercises was when I attended one of Dr. Stephen Chang's workshops. Dr. Chang gave a lecture on the three Animal Exercises, the Crane, Turtle, and Deer. I was amazed at Dr. Chang's findings as to how important these three exercises were for both men and women to do every day. So, as I normally do, since he has given me so many life-changing suggestions, I followed Dr. Chang's recommendation and the results were amazing. When I did the Crane Exercises my digestion was faster and more regular, and my stools were a better consistency (as in fluffy and easy to pass). I also had more energy throughout the day. When I did the Turtle Exercises I felt more relaxed. When I did the Deer Exercises I felt a stronger sexual energy and drive. And the best part? Each exercise took only a minute or less. I cannot thank Dr. Chang enough; he is a very special person in my life. I think he is an amazing, wonderful man, and you will think so, too, when you work these exercises into your daily routine.

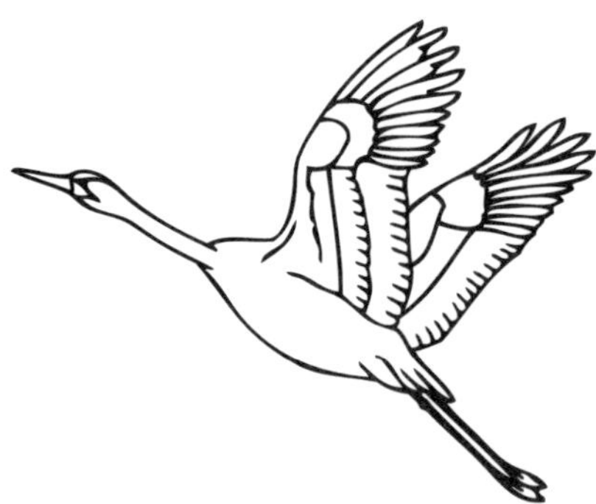

Crane Exercises

The most important of the Crane Exercises is the Stomach Rubbing Exercise, which is what I will be focusing on in this chapter. It is a simple exercise but can have a significant impact in battling weight problems and obesity, as well as in helping cure various stomach ailments and diseases.

Obesity and being overweight are responsible for an astonishing array of health problems in the human body. In addition to the more well-known consequences of elevated weight, such as heart disease, diabetes, cancer, and stroke, being overweight can adversely affect virtually every organ and system in our body: the glandular system and hormones; the digestive system; the lungs, bones, joints, and muscles; the skin; the brain, spinal cord, and other nerves in the nervous system; the immune system; and even the eyes—among many other previously unheard of effects. It can cause health problems ranging from hair loss to sexual dysfunction to slow wound healing to birth defects.

In addition, weight gain becomes harder to manage as we get older. We gain weight more easily, and our body proportions change as hormones change. One of these changes is that fat deposits more in the abdomen than the extremities, for both men and women. The stomach rubbing exercise is ideal for combating both the issues of abdominal weight gain and of health problems due to weight gain.

Begin by lying down flat on your back and relaxing (note that all of the exercises in this chapter can be done lying down, sitting, or standing). Next, put the palm of your hand on your navel, using your right if you're right-handed or left if you're left-handed. Now start rubbing clockwise from the center—that is, starting on your right-hand side and moving to the left. Begin in small circles and then gradually enlarge the circles until you are rubbing the upper and lower edges of your abdomen (see following figures). You don't need to press down with any force; only apply a slight pressure, and rub slowly.

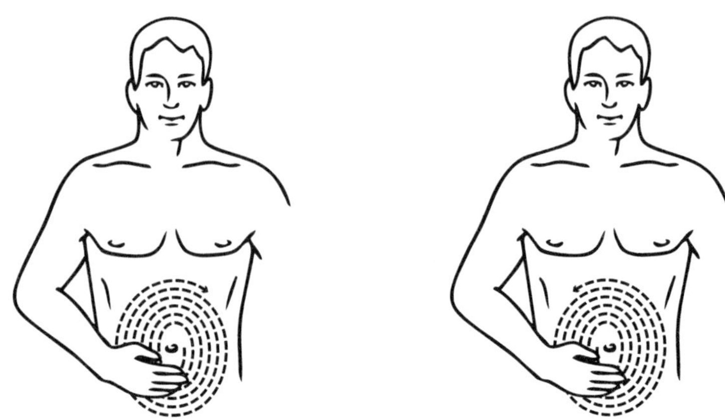

FIGURE 84.
Crane Stomach Rubbing Exercise showing clockwise and counter-clockwise directions.

Once you have completed the above exercise, reverse it. Begin in the center again, but this time rub in a counter-clockwise direction (left to right). Repeat both the clockwise and counter-clockwise exercises as many times as you wish. Personally I do nine circles in each direction, clockwise and counter-clockwise, every day.

An alternate, brisker version of the Stomach Rubbing Exercise can also be done. Begin by rubbing the palms of your hands together vigorously and then placing them, palms down, on your abdomen, on either side of your navel. Now rub both sides of your abdomen briskly, following the arrows shown in the next figure; both hands should be in sync, meeting near the navel on the down-swing. Keep rubbing until the friction heats up your abdominal tissues. You may repeat as many times as you wish. Because this version of the exercise brings more stimulation and energy to your abdomen than the previous version, it can more effectively be used for diseases of the internal organs, peristaltic problems, and abdominal weight loss.

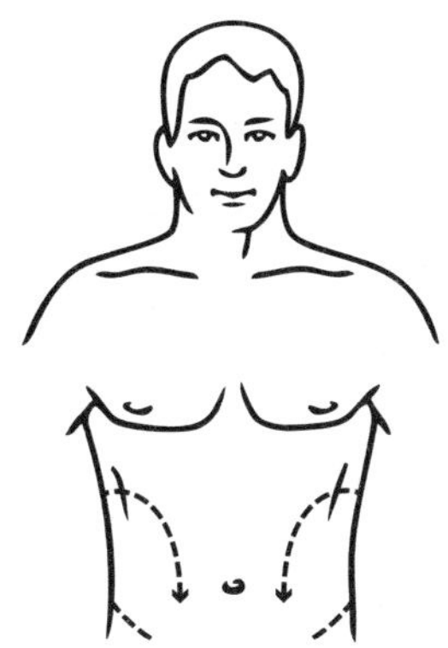

FIGURE 85.
An alternate Stomach Rubbing Exercise.

I recommend using your powers of visualization and imagination during these exercises. Feel the energy coming from your hands and penetrating into the skin and organs underneath. Feel the energy being retained and heating up your abdominal tissues. As more energy penetrates your body, the area around your navel will begin to burn as if a fire had been started within it. Focus on this feeling every time you perform these exercises.

Dr. Chang has had many patients come to him with amazing healings from performing these simple Stomach Rubbing Exercises. He recommends rubbing in a clockwise direction if constipation is the difficulty, and counter-clockwise if a person is suffering from diarrhea. He has heard from patients who suffered from chronic constipation and diarrheal conditions for years who were quickly cured once they started using these techniques. He recommends both directions to help heal stomach ulcers.

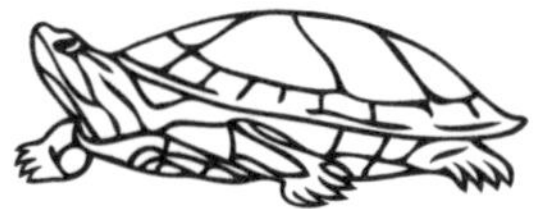

Turtle Exercises

The origin of the Turtle Exercises comes from an ancient Taoist story of a family trapped in a cave who had a dwindling food supply and little water. When they observed the motions of a turtle they found in the cave, they modeled his subtle neck extensions and contractions, because he had been able to survive on almost nothing. Legend has it the family was not found until many years later, subsisting as the turtle had on only a few drops of water and using only spare head and neck movements.

This parable emphasizes the importance of exercising the neck, a vital part of our body that connects our head, the center of our being, with our body. The Turtle Exercise stretches, stimulates, and energizes all the nerves of the neck, which forms the pathway for nerves that lead from the brain to the rest of our central nervous system throughout our body. If you can gain control over this complex of nerves, you can control the entire functioning of your body.

The Turtle Exercise stretches the entire spine, energizes the neck, strengthens the shoulder muscles, and removes fatigue, stiffness, and soreness from the neck and shoulder muscles. In addition, the thyroid and parathyroid glands are stimulated and strengthened, which improves the body's metabolism. Performing the Turtle Exercise on a daily basis will leave you feeling younger and radiating an inner beauty, a result of the proper functioning of your inner energy systems.

The Turtle Exercise may be done standing, sitting, or lying down, though I prefer to do it in the sitting position. I recommend doing this exercise when you wake up in the morning, and also just before you go to sleep at night. You may also perform it whenever you feel tension or tightness in your neck, upper back, or shoulders.

First, stand or sit looking straight ahead with your back straight. I recommend either looking at a soft, muted light or keeping your eyes gently closed. Keep your body relaxed and your fingers clasped around your thumbs as you make a fist (this hand lock prevents energy from spilling out through the fingers). Now, slowly lower your chin to your chest, while at the same time stretching the top of your head upward (see figure)—hold for about one second.

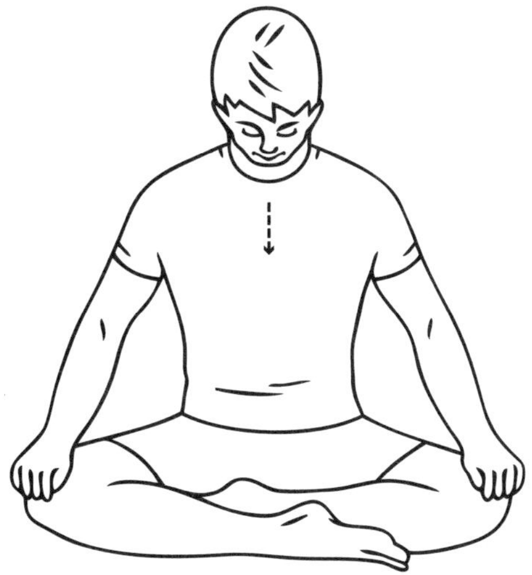

FIGURE 86. The Turtle Exercise, step one.

Slowly inhale as you execute this motion and position. The back of your neck should feel an upward pull, and your shoulders should relax downward.

Next, slowly tilt your head backward as far as it will go (see figure) for about one second. Slowly exhale as you do this movement. Your chin should be pulled upward, and your throat should be slightly stretched. Both shoulders should also be pulled upward while you do this, as if you were trying to touch them to your ears. Repeat this cycle of both positions for a total of 12 times. Make sure you do not force the movements.

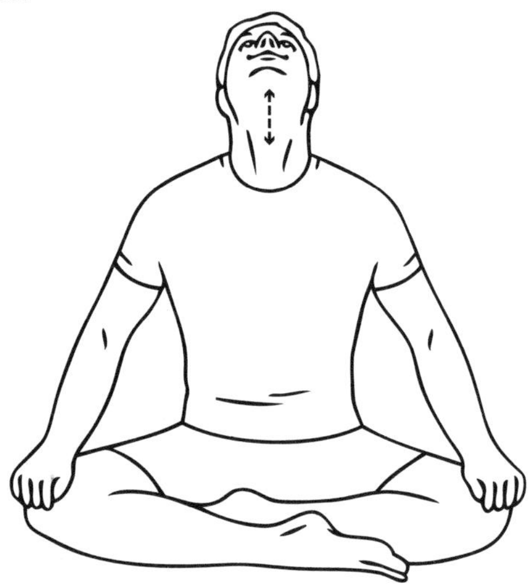

FIGURE 87. The Turtle Exercise, step two.

Remember to focus on what you are doing. If your mind wanders, practice the Power of the Mind (see Chapter 19) and bring it back. Have patience in practicing this exercise, and I believe it will lead you to a treasure of healthful, emotional, and spiritual benefits, as it has for me.

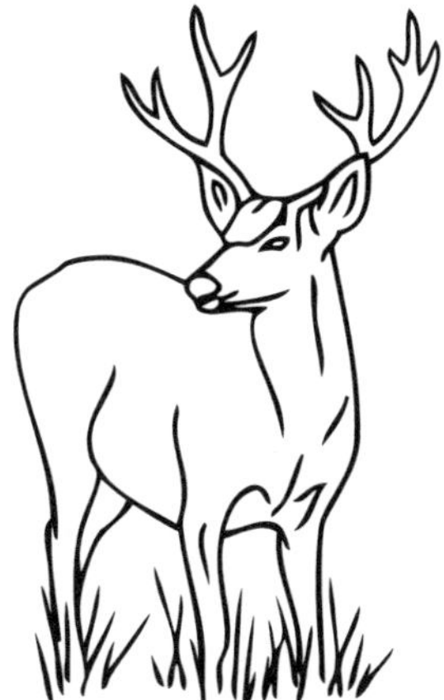

Deer Exercises

In ancient times, Taoist sages noticed the deer for its strong sexual and reproductive abilities. Thus the Deer Exercises were designed, for both men and women, to enhance the reproductive organs, reproductive ability, sexual performance and the sexual experience.

Male

For the male, there are four important objectives and benefits in performing the male Deer Exercise: (1) It builds up the tissues of the sexual organs, (2) It draws energy up through six of the seven glands of the body into the pineal gland to elevate spirituality, (3) Self-determination, and (4) It builds up sexual ability and enables the man to prolong intercourse. The Deer Exercise enables a man to pump semen out of the prostate in small doses during orgasm (pumping it in the other direction into other glands and blood vessels), thus prolonging intercourse.

The Deer Exercises may be done standing, sitting, or lying down. As with all Taoist exercises, focus on what you are doing and put other thoughts out of your mind. Concentrate on the purpose of the physical motions and feel the effects in your body. This will enhance the results and unify your body and mind to bring full power to the purpose.

It is best to do this exercise without clothing on. First, rub your palms together vigorously, creating heat between your palms. Next, cup your testicles with your right hand so that the palm of your hand completely covers them. Do not squeeze, just maintain a light pressure. Place the palm of your left hand on your groin area, one inch below your navel (see figure).

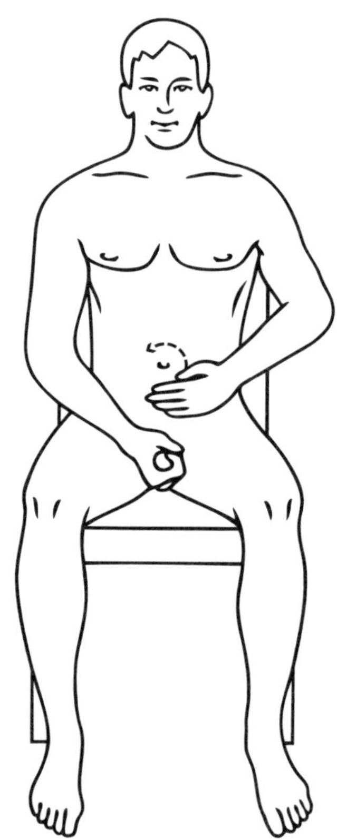

FIGURE 88. Deer Exercise for the male.

With a slight pressure so that a gentle warmth begins to build in the area of your pubis, move your left hand in clockwise or counter-clockwise circles (small, about 3 to 4 inches in diameter) 81 times. Vigorously rub your hands together again. Now switch hands so that your left hand cups your testicles and your right hand is on your groin. Repeat the circular rubbing in the opposite direction of where you started, 81 times.

Do the second exercise when you wake up in the morning as well as before you go to sleep at night. Begin by tightening the muscles around your anus and drawing them up and in. If you are doing it properly it will feel as if air is being drawn up your rectum, or as if your entire anal area is being drawn in and upward. Tighten as hard as you can and hold as long as you are able to do so comfortably. In the beginning try to hold for at least one second. Now pause and relax. Repeat the anal contractions as many times as you can without feeling discomfort, pausing in between. As you do this, concentrate on feeling a tingling sensation (similar to an electric shock) ascend up your spine, similar to goose bumps.

In the beginning you may only be able to hold the anal sphincter muscles tight for a few seconds. However, continue the exercise regularly, and after several weeks you will be able to hold the muscles tight for quite a while—experts can hold for minutes—without experiencing fatigue or strain. Once you can go longer, you may experience a natural high upon performing this exercise. This arises because tightening the anus puts pressure on the prostate gland, which stimulates it to secrete hormones such as endorphins. When the prostate goes into spasms, a small orgasm is experienced and a natural high is produced.

To determine whether or not the second Deer Exercise is having an effect on the prostate gland, try the urination test. As you urinate, try to stop the stream of urine entirely through anal muscle contractions. If you are able to do so, then you are doing the exercise properly and it is achieving its purpose.

The Deer Exercises can correct many sexual problems such as premature ejaculation, low sex hormone levels, infections of the testicles, wet dreams, and impotence. They may help prevent these problems from occurring as well. In addition, they are good for overall healing because they build up general immunity against disease-causing agents.

Bear in mind that the Deer Exercises for the male are physical, mental, and spiritual. They improve one's sexual abilities as it builds up the energy reserves in the body. Over time, the mental processes are heightened as well, and the result is often a growing feeling of inner tranquility. This mental tranquility is a necessary prerequisite for the development of one's spirituality as well.

Female

As I discuss in Chapter 14, Strengthening the Reproductive Organs, I believe it is preferable to stop menstruation in order to strengthen the female reproductive system, which you can achieve by regularly performing the female Deer Exercises. In the Taoist tradition, uterine blood is meant specifically to nourish a developing fetus in the womb and afterward to support breastfeeding. If a woman is not pregnant or breastfeeding, menstrual blood represents a depletion of energy and vitality.

An additional benefit of these exercises is that difficulties with menstruation—such as emotional swings, water retention, hormone blockages, cramps, and abnormal flow of blood—can be eliminated. Further, the exercises trigger the enhancement of estrogen production. If you are approaching or in menopause, estrogen will be spread throughout your reproductive system and can greatly relieve the symptoms of menopause. This is preferable to hormone supplements since the body naturally balances the amount to how much it needs, which changes from hour to hour. The vagina also benefits from these exercises, becoming tighter, meatier, and more flexible.

Do the female Deer Exercises in the morning when you wake up and at night before you go to sleep.

In the first exercise, sit slightly cross-legged on the floor, in such a way that the heel of one foot rests against the opening of your vagina (see figure). Keep a steady and firm pressure against the clitoris, which may create a pleasant sensation due to the stimulation of the genital area and the subsequent release of sexual energy. If you are not able to place your foot in the position described, use a fairly hard, round object such as a baseball against the vaginal opening.

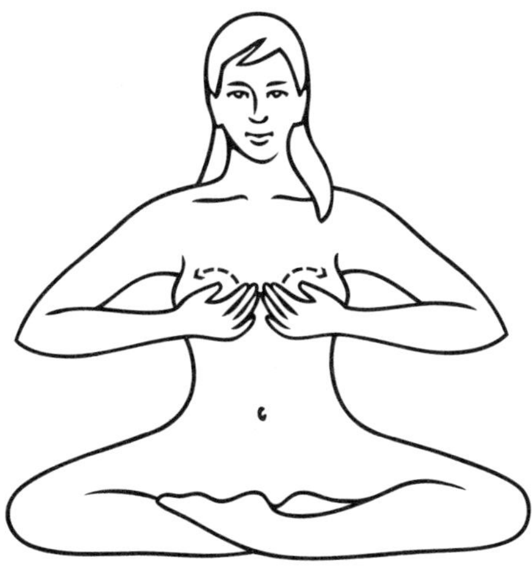

FIGURE 89. Deer Exercise for the female.

Now, vigorously rub your hands together, creating heat. Then place your hands on your breasts so that you feel the heat from your hands enter into the skin (see preceding figure). Rub your breasts slowly in an outward, circular motion, moving your right hand counter-clockwise and your left hand clockwise. Rub in this circular manner for a minimum of 36 times or a maximum of 360 times, up to two times per day. Once you have succeeded in stopping your period, it is not necessary to do 360 hand rotations. At this point less than 100 rotations, twice a day, should be sufficient to maintain a suspension of menstruation. If you choose to resume menstruation, simply cease this exercise.

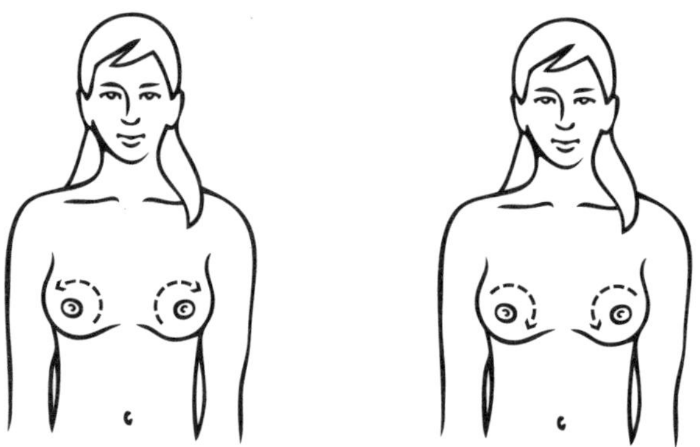

FIGURE 90.
Dispersion is shown on the left, and stimulation is shown on the right.

Rubbing the breasts in an outward circular motion is called "dispersion" and may help prevent lumps and cancer of the breast. It may also decrease the size of breasts that are too large and flabby. Conversely, rubbing in the opposite direction, called "stimulation," has the opposite effect and enlarges undersized breasts (see figures above).

Try to avoid touching your nipples when you do the above

exercise as many women's nipples are very sensitive and easily overstimulated. An increase in nipple sensitivity will result if the exercise is being done correctly.

The second exercise can be done either sitting or lying down. First, tighten the muscles of your vagina and anus as if you were trying to close both openings, and then try to draw your rectum upward inside your body, further contracting your anal muscles. This should feel as if air is being drawn up into your rectum and vagina. Hold these muscles tight for as long as you can without discomfort. You may insert a finger into your vagina when you do the contractions to determine the strength of your contractions and to monitor development over time. Relax, and then repeat the anal and vaginal contractions. Repeat as many times as you wish.

The first few anal and vaginal contractions may be hard to do and maintain. Eventually, however, you will be able to increase the number of times you can do it as well as the length of time you are able to hold the contractions. When done properly, a pleasant feeling will travel from the base of your anus through your spinal column to the top of your head.

You should also massage and stimulate the lips of your vagina during both Deer Exercises. Rub the lips and be sure to apply pressure to each point in the figure shown below.

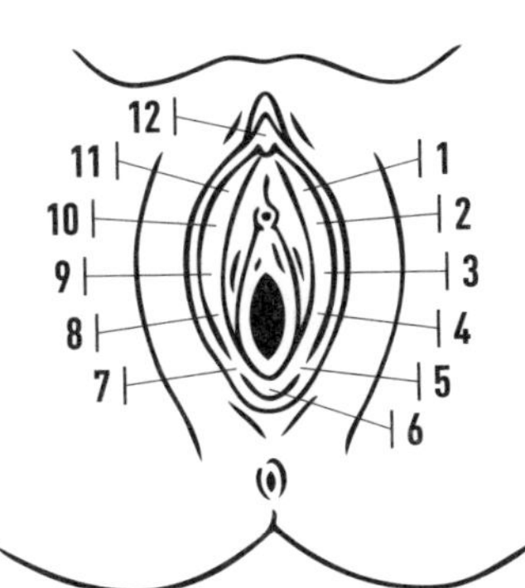

FIGURE 91. Acupressure points surrounding the vaginal opening.

The method of massaging the vaginal opening is flexible and can include a partner. In the first exercise, sitting on your heel or a baseball achieves stimulation. Alternatively, you can rub one breast at a time and rub your lips with your free hand, making sure to press each pressure point. It is very beneficial if your partner rubs your vagina, because the energy that flows through your partner's hands flows into your body. Another method is to have your partner rub your breasts while you rub or press your vagina with your hand.

Remember, you can do any of these three Animal Exercises anytime or anywhere during the day, in just 60 seconds.

For more information on the exercises mentioned in this chapter, go to:
www.DOITORAGEQUICKLY.com
www.JBBERNS.com

14

STRENGTHENING THE REPRODUCTIVE ORGANS: PROSTATE MASSAGE/EJACULATION CONTROL AND STOPPING MENSTRUATION

For 60 Seconds:
For men, massage your prostate and monitor ejaculation; for women, perform Deer Exercises

Energy equals life. Every day there is a rough balance of energy in and out of our bodies. Little by little we are depleted of our energy as we age. We must protect this most precious gift! In this chapter I will discuss how you can do just that by exercising your reproductive organs. The first exercise I recommend is the prostate massage, which will help keep a man's prostate healthy into his old age. The second is the practice of ejaculation control, which prevents a man's energy from flowing out on a regular basis. The third is a surprisingly simple exercise for women to halt menstruation, which has a similar effect to ejaculation control as men as it keeps energy from flowing out.

In my own experience, I have felt my body slow down (overall health and power, sexually and health-wise) after I was 30 years old. By applying and doing the prostate massage, it has made me feel younger and increased my sex drive. As far as ejaculation control, I have realized that my sexual performance has increased by not emitting so often (following the recommendations listed in this chapter), and my sensitivity as a lover has also increased. Although the prostate massage and ejaculation control have been a very difficult sell to some of my close male friends, the ones who were open-minded and performed both have thanked me in spades, along with a few free dinners.

Prostate Massage

I recommend, for men north of 30 years old, to at least once a week, preferably in the shower, perform the prostate massage (I discuss the how-to in detail below). The reason I am recommending this to you, as do my Eastern medicine mentor Dr. Stephen Chang and most Taoist masters, is that giving yourself a prostate massage will keep your prostate soft and supple. This is the man's furnace that so-called "heats the house:" you need to attend to it. We clean our teeth, our ears, our armpits, our nose, and so on. What many men don't realize is that they should also be cleaning their anal cavity as well, which the prostate massage also accomplishes. This is a foreign concept to most Westerners, but it is a necessity for all men.

In my opinion, most men have prostate problems because their prostate is not soft and supple, and at times it is under- or overused. A good analogy for the prostate is that it is similar to a washer pump in a car. If you don't use the pump, it will dry up. However, if you overuse it, it will seize up. There needs to be a balance of how much you use your "pump."

To the men out there, trust me, you need to do this for yourselves. By the time most men are north of 50 years old they have an enlarged prostate. Performing the prostate massage will keep your prostate at its natural size, not enlarged, which would push against the bladder and cause frequent untimely urination or the sensation that you have to urinate. I prefer that you perform the prostate massage instead of taking a biopharmaceutical that could have drastic side effects to your overall well-being. As a very popular sports marketing and sneaker company logo says, "Just do it." You will thank me in later years.

Prostate massage, when performed on a regular basis, has been shown to be good for prostate health in general, and may decrease the risk of prostate enlargement (known as benign prostate hypertrophy, or BPH) and possibly prostate cancer. Studies suggest that BPH, infertility, and chronic prostatitis can all benefit from this practice. The prostate is more likely to become infected or cancerous when blood flow is constricted from muscular tension and lack of stimulation. In the Far East, prostate massage has been used for centuries to maintain the health of the gland and improve sexual health in general.

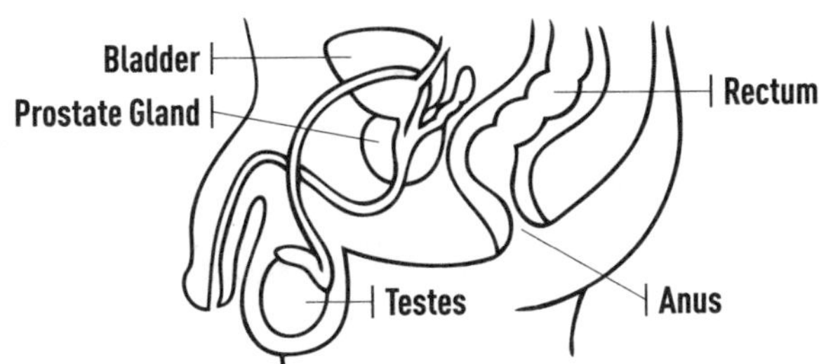

FIGURE 92. Side view of the male reproductive system.

Performing prostate massage is relatively simple for a man to do himself. You may want to urinate or do a bowel movement before the massage so you feel as relaxed as possible. Be sure to wipe your anus before you insert your finger, as this part of the body is unclean. In addition, make sure your fingernails are clean and smooth, and wash your hands thoroughly. The massage can be performed standing or squatting. It is done simply by inserting your finger inside your anus and reaching back and up toward your navel until you feel your prostate gland (see figures below). You do not have to push in too far, just around an inch and a half. Insert gently, as the rectal skin is fragile.

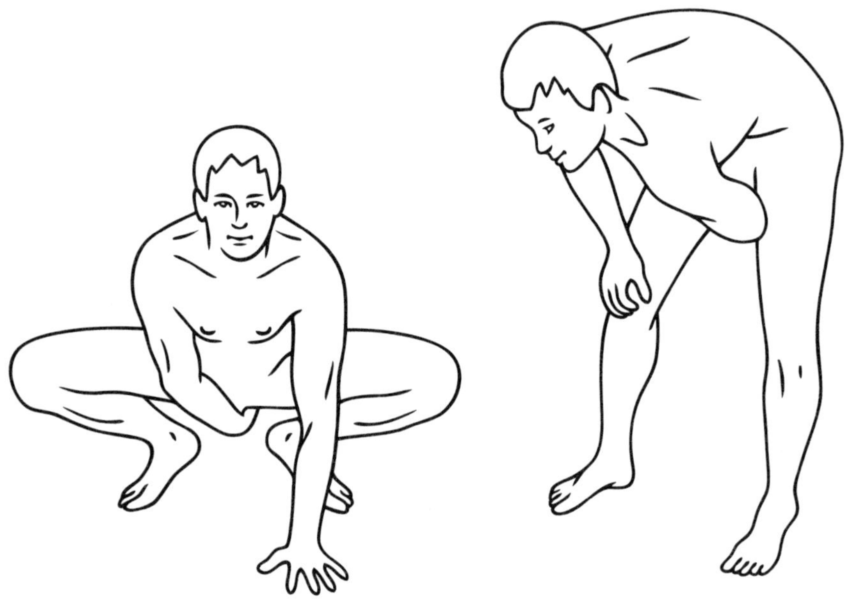

FIGURE 93. Two possible positions in which to perform the prostate massage.

The prostate gland is a small, round bulb of tissue about the size of a large walnut. Give it a gentle massage by rubbing it along its sides, then rub on the gland's central portion (don't use too much pressure here, as this is where some sensitive nerves are located); in general, rub as hard as possible without causing pain (usually around 10 seconds). Do not touch the prostate gland with your fingernails. You may have the sensation of having to urinate even though you don't have to; this is normal.

Using a little lubricant will make insertion easier. If you do, I recommend that you use lubricant made of natural ingredients, as the lining of the rectum is quite permeable. Personally, I use and recommend Royal Jade Cream (see the end of this chapter for purchasing information). The following ingredients should be avoided, as they are known to be toxic and may be, or are known to be, carcinogenic:

- FD & C Blue #1
- P-hydroxyanisole
- Triethanlolamine (TEA)
- Diethanolamine (DEA)
- Iron oxide
- Lead acetate
- Toluene
- Dibutyl phthalate
- Acetone
- EDTA
- PVP
- BHT
- BNPD
- Coal tar
- Phenol
- Sodium saccharin
- Sodium carrageenan

You can also have a partner perform the prostate massage for you, which can increase the pleasure. Just make sure the person follows all of the guidelines above. Gloves are an option, although not necessary if the person's nails are smooth and his or her hands have been washed.

Some men have reservations about doing prostate massage

because they think of it as a "dirty" part of their body or have anxiety about the massage being a homosexual act. Firstly, there is nothing dirty about the human body; it is only our mind that tells us this. Secondly, it's a preference for the same gender that makes a person homosexual; a massage is not going to convert anyone. And thirdly, your health is more important than either of these issues. Your overall prostate health should benefit, and you will also be able to monitor the area for any changes in texture or size that could indicate a health issue that needs attention.

Ejaculation Control for Men

Diet, exercise, and sexual discipline are three fundamental practices of Taoist health and longevity regimens. It is thought that the ejaculation of semen not only represents a loss of vital resources, but a loss of spiritual energy as well. Depending on your age and state of health and vigor, there is a rough maximum of ejaculations you should follow daily, weekly, yearly, and even seasonally. It is believed that this practice is responsible for many men living to be one hundred years old and beyond.

Semen is made up of sperm, which are suspended in a fluid called seminal plasma. Sperm are made in the testicles and mature in the epididymis. The fluids in seminal plasma come from different glands in the man's body: the seminal vesicles and the prostate and bulbourethral glands. Semen is composed of proteins, amino acids, sugars, prostaglandins, enzymes, acids, and vitamins and minerals. If ejaculation is suppressed (not the sexual act, only the final ejaculation), at least part of the ejaculatory is preserved such that those bodily resources are not wasted. Further, a sense of fatigue, emptiness, and disinterest in sex does not come over the person if ejaculation is controlled. As Dr. Steven Chang says in his book *The Tao of Sexology*, "Ejaculation is often called 'coming.' The precise word for it should be 'going,' because everything—the erection, vital energy, millions of live sperms, hormones, nutrients, even a little of the man's personality—goes away. It is a great sacrifice for the man, spiritually, mentally, and physically."

Because the goal of Taoism is to acquire and maintain as much energy as possible and to lose as little as possible, ideally your goal should be to not ejaculate at all. However, if you feel you have to ejaculate, as many men do, I recommend abiding by the Rhythm Theory. Everything in the universe has its rhythms and cycles, and human beings are no exception. In a similar way to women having menstrual cycles, men also have cycles. According to ancient Taoist texts, men have certain time intervals in which they can ejaculate without doing harm to themselves. The idea is that if they wait the appropriate time interval between ejaculations, they will be able to replenish lost vital energy and nutrients.

Roughly, healthy men in their twenties need not be too concerned about the amount they ejaculate. By their thirties, however, men should start conserving. The Rhythm Theory formula is as follows:

Age x 0.2 = Interval to wait between ejaculations (in days)

See the table below for the recommendation for your age. This is just a benchmark. If you really want to stay youthful, ejaculate even less than recommended below. In this way you will preserve your power and use it to heal your body and keep it looking and feeling young. As I said, however, abstaining is best. Following this chart will result in a loss of vital energy, but at least it will help you build up your energy reserves. Also keep in mind that, while no special considerations are necessary for spring or summer, it is thought that a man should conserve more in the fall and avoid ejaculation altogether during the cold of winter.

Age	Days between ejaculations
20	4
30	6
40	8
50	10
60	12
70	14
80	16
90	18
100	20

TABLE 1. Recommended wait-time between ejaculations, depending on age.

In addition to learning to control the frequency of ejaculation, you can also control the amount of semen you ejaculate and learn to "come lightly." For this technique, rather than approaching climax in a frenzy, go slow and savor the release. Then, before the ejaculation is over, squeeze off your urogenital canal with a deep contraction of your anus and penile shaft. Immediately after emission, rhythmically contract your entire urogenital diaphragm for a minute or two with anal sphincter locks. This will tighten up your pelvic floor, which becomes loose and flaccid after ejaculation, and thereby prevents postcoital loss of energy through the perineum, anus, and urogenital canal.

Bear in mind that no one is saying not to have relations.

On the contrary, abstinence would do even more damage. It would deprive you of the therapeutic benefits that sexual stimulation offers. In addition, having no intercourse would create yearning and lead to nocturnal emissions.

Emittance, Men and Women

Women do not have the same issues that men face upon sexual intercourse. For men, orgasm results in depletion, while for women, since they don't "leak," nothing is lost. Their sexual drive is not diminished nor their interest after the first act. Due to these facts of nature, in terms of sexuality, the harmony of the Yin and Yang must be cultivated primarily by men.

A male's body is clearly sexually different from a female's. A woman's capacity to emit for orgasm is inexhaustible, while a man's is not and will slow as the years go by. There is a saying attributed to boxers—don't see the lady before the fight. The idea was that if the boxer saw a woman before his fight and had sexual intercourse with her, he would be weaker the next day, because that is a man's essence, his power to procreate. My friends, I could not feel more strongly about ejaculation control. It takes a tremendous amount of discipline, but in my personal experience, it will make you a better lover and a more sensitive person. Although, at times, I myself can be like a shoemaker going shoeless. It's 99% practice, 1% theory on this issue of ejaculation control.

Menstruation and Strengthening the Female System

I believe it is preferable to stop menstruation if you can to strengthen your reproductive system. This system is composed of the vagina, uterus, ovaries, and the breasts, all of which are inter-related. In the Taoist tradition, uterine blood is meant specifically to nourish a developing fetus in the womb and afterward to support breastfeeding. If a woman is not pregnant or breastfeeding, menstrual blood represents depletion of energy and vitality. In the same way that nourishment and energy is thought to be depleted when men ejaculate, so it is with menstrual blood in a woman.

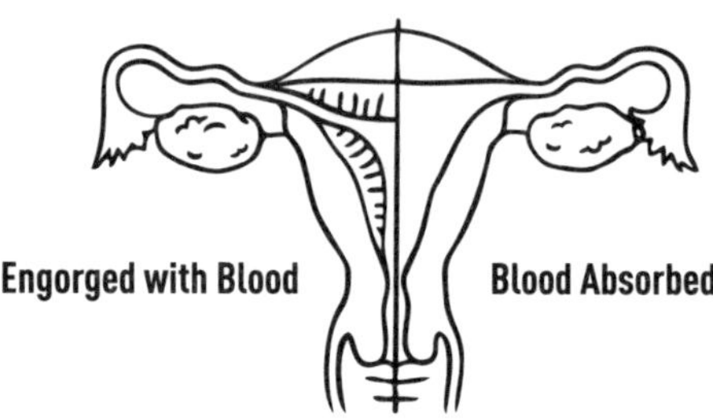

FIGURE 94. The female reproductive system, showing the uterus during menstruation (left) and when a woman is not menstruating (right).

You can cease menstruation through the disciplined practice of Deer Exercises for women (find detailed instructions in Chapter 13, Animal Exercises). If it is done properly and more than the recommended minimum of 36 hand rotations twice a day, up to 360 times twice a day, you can stop menstruation completely. Your body will rush blood to your breasts rather than your uterus, and your body will react just as though a baby is nursing regularly. Menstrual irregularities such as cramps will also be corrected, and sexual ability will be enhanced.

Note that it is important to focus and not let your mind wander during the exercises. This includes not letting it become sexually stimulating, as it will be for many. It may take only two weeks to six months to cease menstruation, or for some women up to a year.

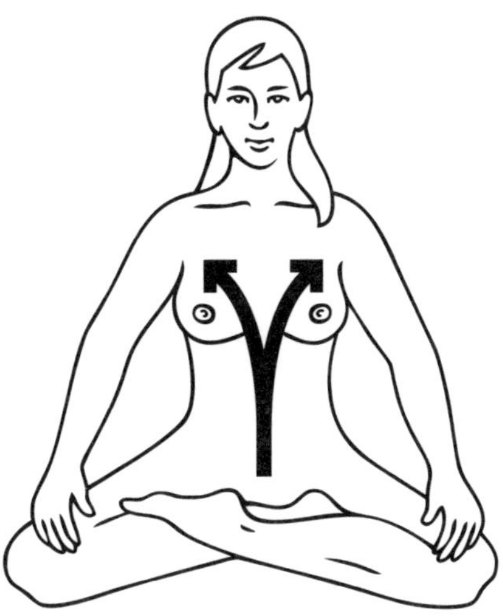

FIGURE 95. Strengthening the female system.

Taoists refer to this practice as "turning back the clock" because it re-energizes the entire body, especially the sexual organs. In fact, regular application of the Deer Exercises are thought to preserve beauty in women and stop the physical aging process from the time the exercises begin. However, it is not expected to extend the fertile period, and menopause will fall at its expected time, albeit without the usual attendant problems most experience.

Exercise your reproductive organs, and turn back the clock.

For more information on strengthening your reproductive system and Royal Jade Cream, go to:
www.DOITORAGEQUICKLY.com
www.JBBERNS.com

15
ESSENTIAL STRETCHES

For 60 Seconds:
Stretch.

Many times the most important things we can do for our health and well-being are the simplest and most natural. Stretching, something we instinctually do for relief when we're tired or stiff, is one of those things. This easy, refreshing practice can have tremendous benefits if you incorporate it into your daily routine.

Stretching is beneficial for people of all ages. When you stretch regularly, you're able to increase your range of motion, moving your limbs and joints further than you would be able to otherwise. In addition, the further you are able to stretch, the further you can move your limbs and joints before an injury occurs. Post-exercise stretching can also help speed or eliminate workout recovery time, decrease muscle soreness, and help ensure that muscles and tendons are in good working order.

As we age, stretching becomes particularly vital. Activities that were once easy become strained, such as tying a shoe, picking up something off the floor, reaching for a high shelf, or zipping a back zipper. Posture can become hunched, altering appearance and putting pressure on internal organs. If you maintain a daily stretching routine, your muscles will remain lengthened and much more flexible, and you can greatly slow this inevitable deterioration. Studies suggest that this is true for arteries as well, and this increased arterial elasticity is beneficial to the circulatory system.

Stretching, done properly, also helps relax tense muscles that have resulted from stress. The feeling of relaxation brings a sense of well-being and relief from tension. Your body will feel great all over after your stretching is completed. In this way stretching benefits your mood and mind as well as your physical health (which is of course also indirectly affected by your mood and your mind).

The great thing is, as with all of my recommendations, a stretching routine requires very little time commitment out of your day.

Here is a summary of some of the many benefits of stretching:

- Reduced muscle tension
- Increased range of movement in the joints
- Decreased muscular injury
- Enhanced muscular coordination
- Increased blood circulation
- Increased energy levels
- Increased flexibility
- Improved posture
- Reduction or prevention of lower back pain
- Relief from pain
- Relaxation and stress relief
- Greater sense of well-being

Below is my list of stretches that you should perform every day (instructions and diagrams to follow).

1. Hamstring and heel stretch
2. Hip circles
3. Arm meditation stretch
4. Lateral hip stretch
5. Angle stretch
6. Horse stance/spine stretch
7. Butterfly stretch
8. Forward bend
9. Extensor stretch
10. Straddle/groin stretch

It is important to do the stretches when your body is already warm, such as after a shower (when I like to do them) or after lightly exercising. Stretching cold muscles is like stretching a cold rubber band: it could snap. To prevent injuries, always remember to stretch when your body is already warmed up.

You should hold all of these stretches for four to eight seconds each. Don't bounce, but ease slowly into the stretch and hold it. Stretch until you feel a slight, mild tension. As you hold the stretch, the feeling of tension should diminish. If it doesn't, or the tension increases or becomes painful, back off into a more comfortable stretch. Remember, you are stretching, not exercising. You don't need to push it. Stretching is a mild, gentle activity. Breathe slowly and deeply—don't hold your breath. Pay attention to how each stretch feels, and relax while you concentrate on that area being stretched. Everyone is different in their ability to stretch and your own body is different every day, so let it guide you by how the stretch feels.

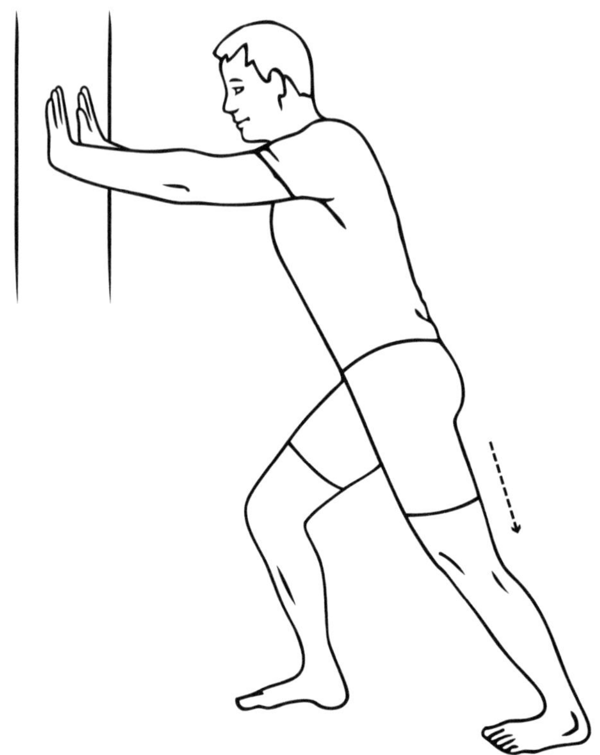

FIGURE 96. Hamstring and heel stretch.

1. Hamstring and Heel Stretch

This stretch is wonderful for the hamstrings (the muscles in the upper backs of your legs). Lean forward and push your hands against a wall. Now lengthen your stance, bending one leg forward while extending the other leg straight behind, while pushing against the wall (see figure above). Keep your back leg straight with your heel flat on the ground, then switch legs.

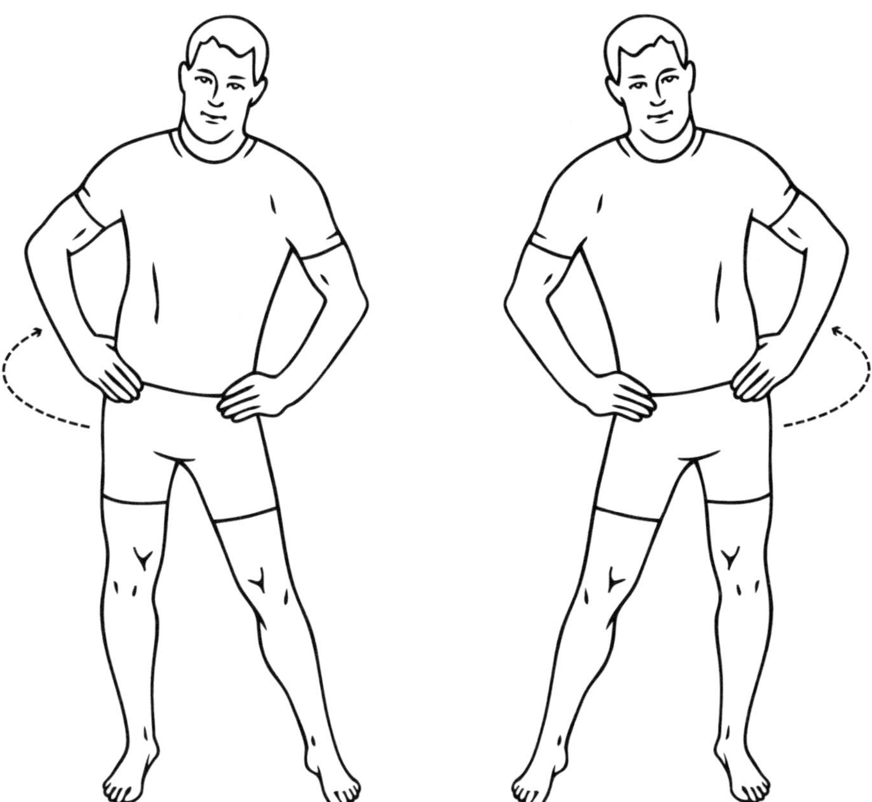

FIGURE 97. Hip circles clockwise and counter-clockwise.

2. Hip Circles

This is a great stretch for the hips. Rotate your hips in a clockwise and then counter-clockwise position, creating a circular movement. Rotate in large circles, big hula-hoop circles.

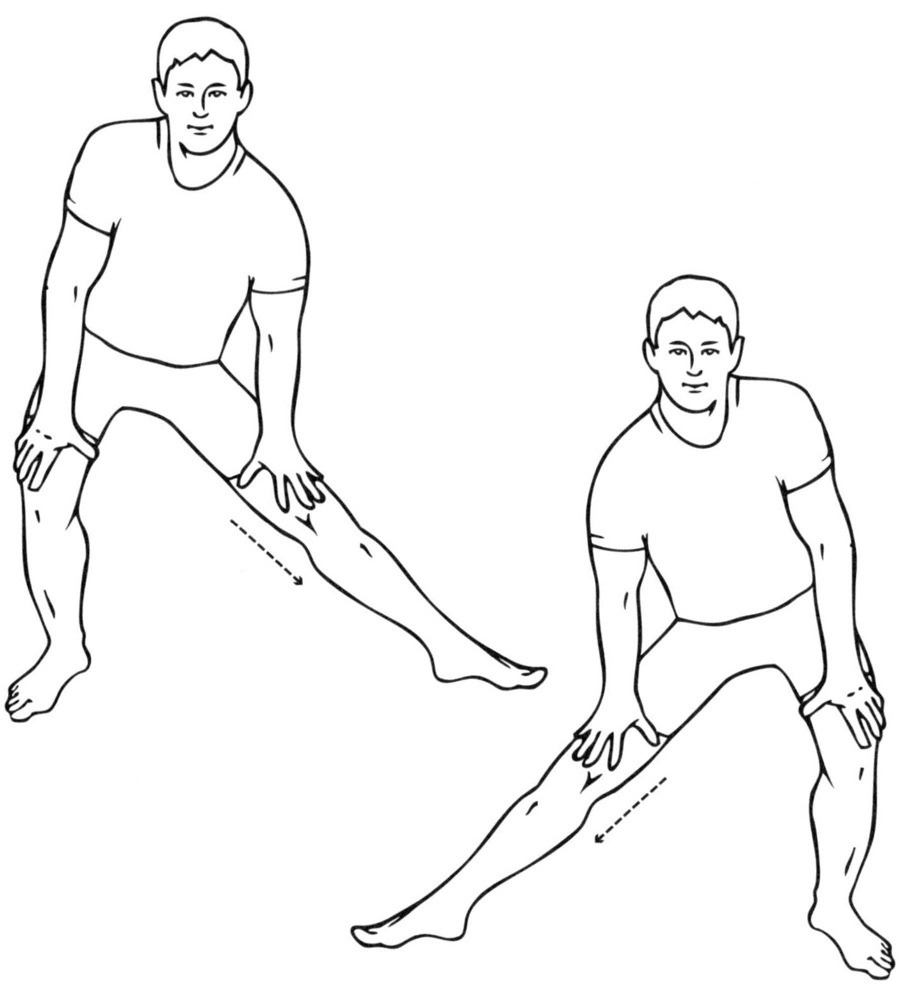

FIGURE 98. Lateral hip stretches to the right and to the left.

3. Lateral Hip Stretch

This is another wonderful stretch for the hips. Stand with your legs wide apart. Bend your right leg first, pointing your knee to the right, letting your left leg fall straight, and gently sway to the right side, pushing your right hand on your right knee. Then repeat on the other side.

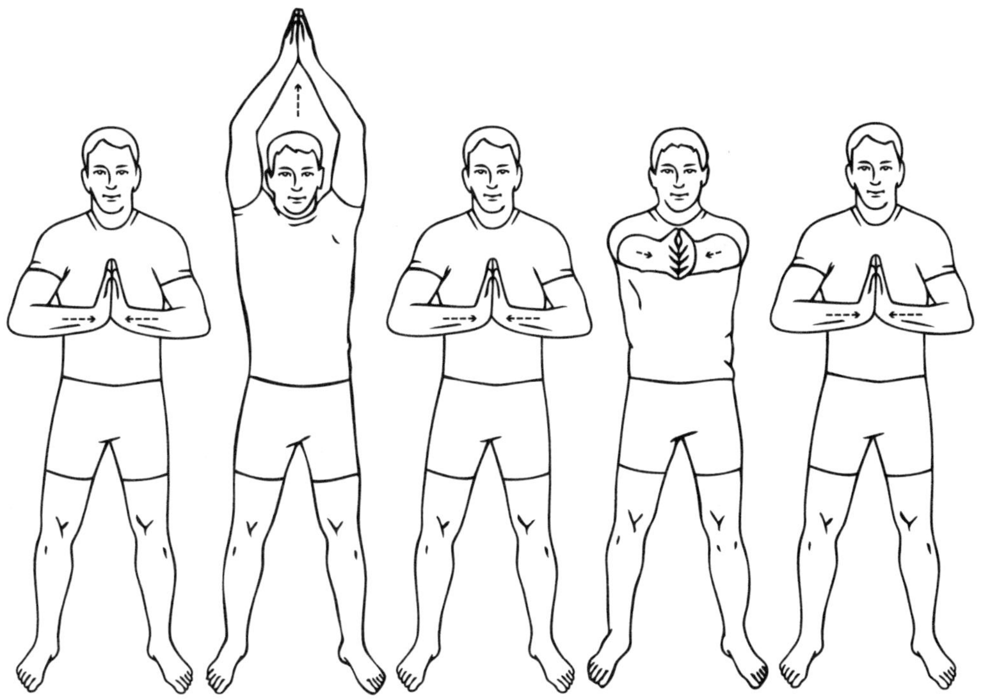

FIGURE 99. For the arm stretch, follow the sequence above.

4. Arm Meditation Stretch

This is a wonderful stretch for the arms and for increasing lung capacity. Begin in a praying position as shown in the figure, with both hands pushing against each other in the center of your chest. Next, raise both arms above your head as you exhale; then bring both arms down to a praying position again as you inhale; then move your hands forward while exhaling (as shown); and finally move your arms back to the starting praying position with an inhale.

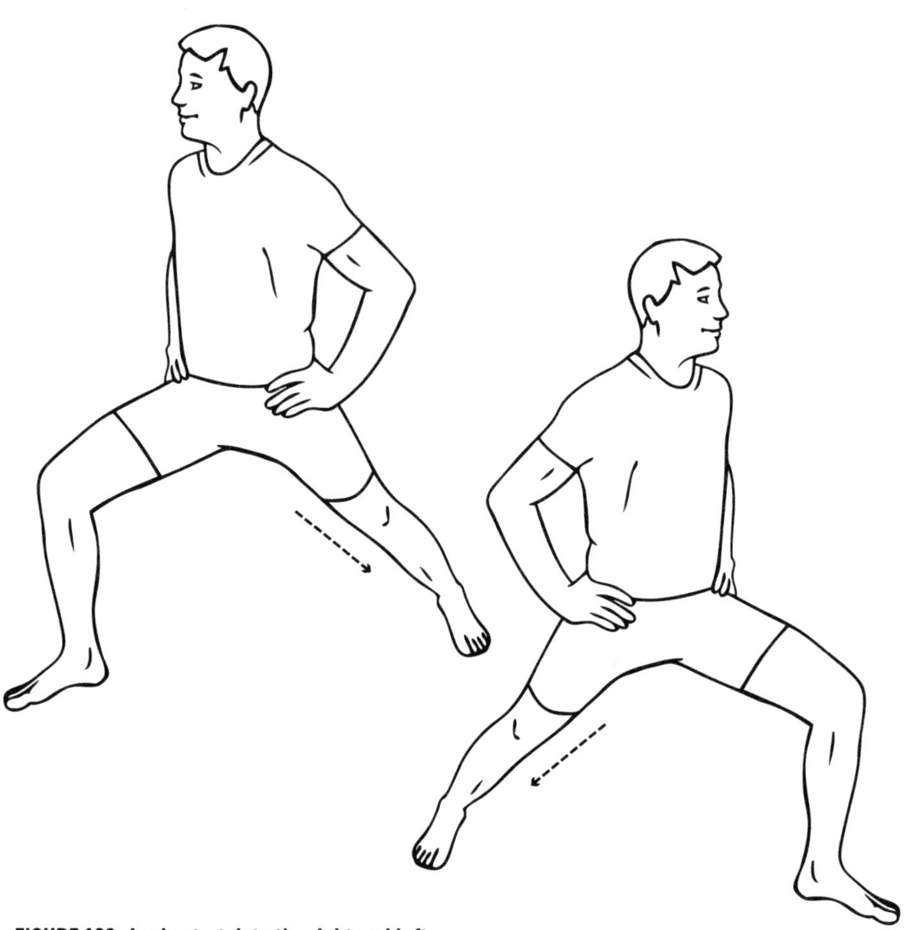

FIGURE 100. Angle stretch to the right and left.

5. Angle Stretch

I love this stretch for the legs. Place your hands on your hips and take a big step forward with your right leg, bending your right knee forward. Move your body into a lunge with your left leg falling straight behind you. Then repeat with the legs switched.

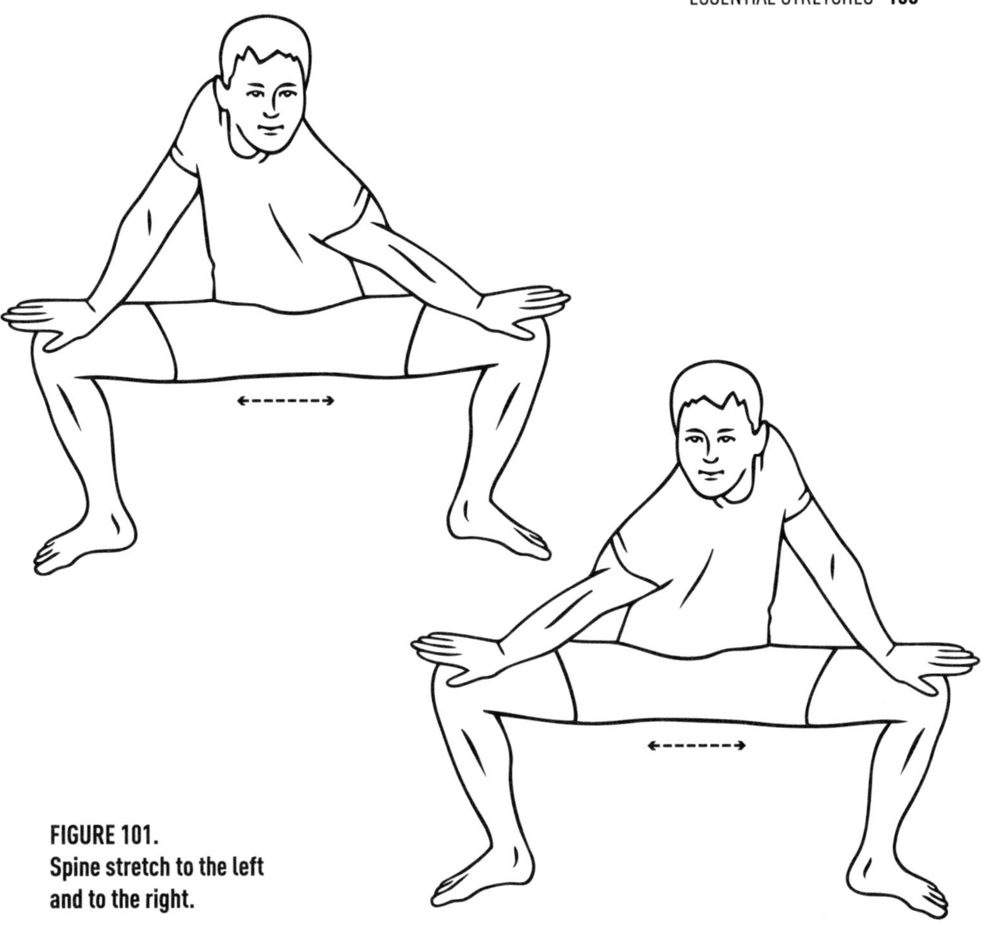

FIGURE 101.
Spine stretch to the left and to the right.

6. Horse Stance/Spine Stretch

I highly recommend this exercise to stretch the spine, groin, and legs. First stand with your legs wide apart, feet turned out as far as they can go. Next, squat as shown in the figure, placing your hands on your knees and letting them have your upper body weight. Squat as far down as you feel comfortable, down to where your thighs are perpendicular to the floor if you can—we call this the horse stance. Now push your right hand against the inner side of your right knee, and twist your right shoulder as far as it will go forward, as shown in the figure. Switch to the other side. Be sure to keep your head straight the entire time.

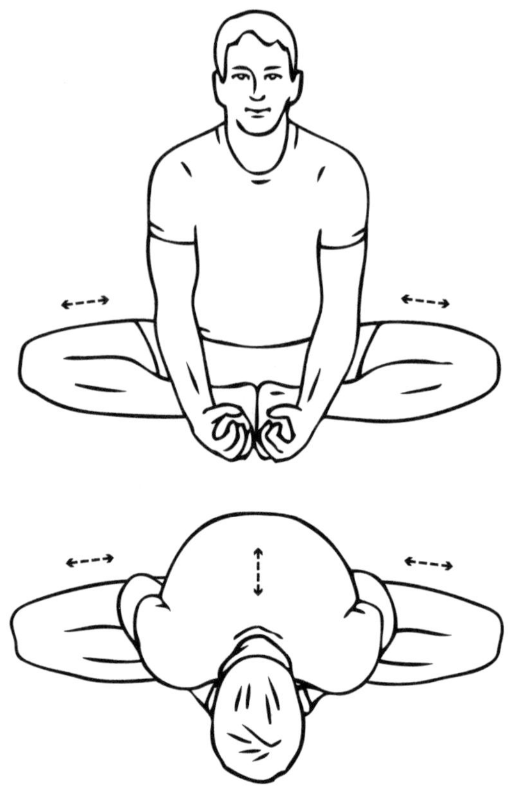

FIGURE 102. Positions of the butterfly stretch.

7. Butterfly Stretch

The butterfly stretch is terrific for the groin and hips. Sitting on the floor with your back straight in an Indian-style position as shown in the figure, try to take the bottoms of both feet and rest them against each other. Then try to pull your knees down to the floor, and bring your head gently forward as far toward the floor as you can go.

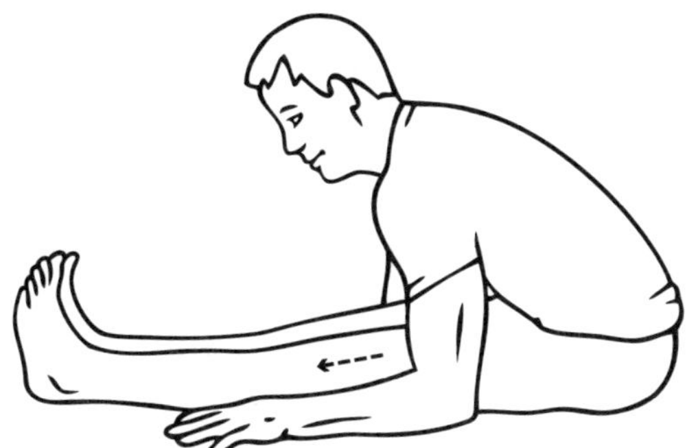

FIGURE 103. Forward bend to stretch the hamstrings.

8. Forward Bend

This stretch is another great one for the hamstrings. Sitting on the floor with both legs together straight in front of you, and your back straight, begin to lean forward. Reach out your hands and grab your toes, and lean down to your legs as far as you can go.

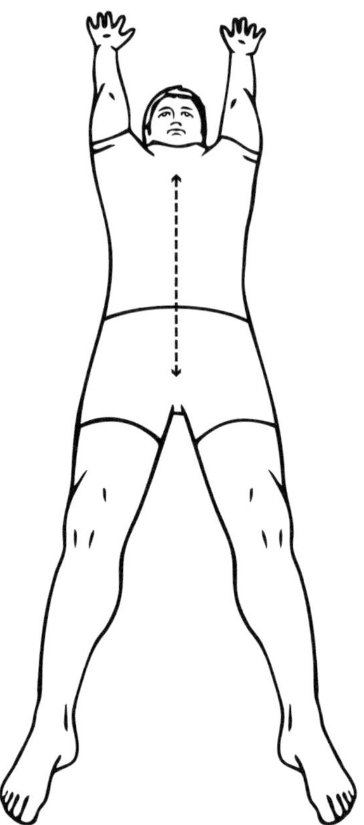

FIGURE 104. Extensor stretch for the entire body and spine (done lying down).

9. Extensor Stretch

This fantastic stretch helps lengthen the entire body and spine. Lie in a supine position (on your back), with both arms straight above your head and both legs straight with both feet pointing, as shown in the figure. Your lower back should be touching the floor, squeezing your abdominal muscles. Extend your body; stretch and lengthen it as far as you can.

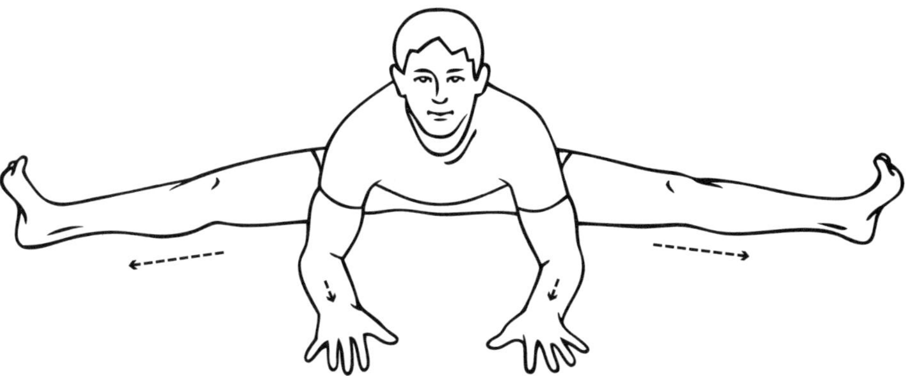

FIGURE 105. Straddle stretch for the groin and hips.

10. Straddle/Groin Stretch

This is a wonderful, and I mean wonderful, stretch for the groin and hips! It is such a very important stretch that I recommend you really take your time with it.

For one minute a day (every day!) rest on the floor in a straddle position with both legs open to the extreme right and left side as shown in the figure above. It's called the splits in gymnastics terms, and if you keep at it you will eventually be able to do it, too. Next, slowly try to bend forward with your back straight, and get as low to the ground as you can. Move your torso over your right leg and press down, then over your left leg and press, then back to center, and press down.

This amazing stretch will open up your hips and increase circulation. As I mentioned in Chapter 1, Correct Posture: Asleep and Awake, our culture dictates that we sit in an upright chair for many of our day-to-day activities, which has the effect of cutting off circulation to our hips and legs. So, to counter this problem, as we cannot sit on the floor during a business dinner or meeting and most public gatherings, the gold nugget is to stretch in this straddle position for at least one minute a day. The result will be better circulation and lymph movement and less throbbing in your hips—and a lower chance of hip replacement in your silver or mature years.

If you would like to see a video demonstration of the stretches described in this chapter as well as others to try, you might want to get my DVD, *The Perfect Martial Arts Workout* (see below for purchasing information).

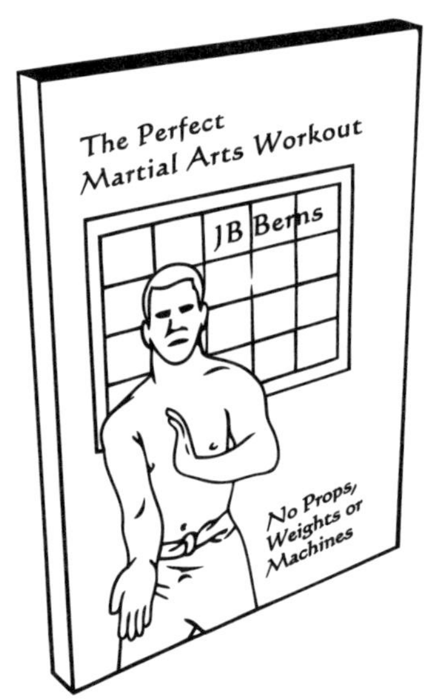

FIGURE 106.
A live demonstration of stretching can be found on my DVD, *The Perfect Martial Arts Workout.*

Let me tell you, the days or mornings that I am rushed and have to make a meeting or for whatever reason cannot get my stretches in, my entire day is out of kilter until I can get to a quiet place and perform my 60-second stretches. When I do not complete my stretches in the morning my body feels unbalanced and tight all over.

My friends, stretching is so important and must, I repeat must, be done every single day of your life. I repeat: every single day of your life, for at least 60 seconds a day. Please, I almost beg you to do so. Your body will feel great all over and you will have increased circulation throughout your entire body. In fact, in my firm opinion and experience, stretching really does prevent injury and relaxes all associated muscles.

For more information on stretching and
***The Perfect Martial Arts Workout* DVD, go to:**
www.DOITORAGEQUICKLY.com
www.JBBERNS.com

16
THE MIRACLE OF REBOUNDING

For 60 Seconds:
Jump on your Urban Rebounder.

The majority of my recommendations in this book do not require expensive, fancy equipment or products, a gym membership, or contraptions that constrain you and bind you to a particular type of activity. In this chapter I would like to tell you about the miracle of rebound exercise. It is an exception to the other chapters in the sense that I ask you to get the Urban Rebounder exercise equipment, but it is still a free-form style of exercise that you can tailor to your needs. The reason I urge you to get this particular piece of equipment is simply because you cannot replicate this exercise in any other way, and it is the best exercise ever created for humans.

Rebounding is done on a soft surface called a rebounder, a sort of miniature trampoline. The device is approximately 30 inches in diameter and around 10 inches off the ground. One jumps on the rebounder vertically, no more than a few inches off of the surface. You can perform aerobics routines, hold weights for a resistance exercise, jog in place, or just bounce to get your heart pumping and lymph flowing. For beginners or those with unstable balance, a stabilizer bar (seen in the following figure) can be used to hold onto.

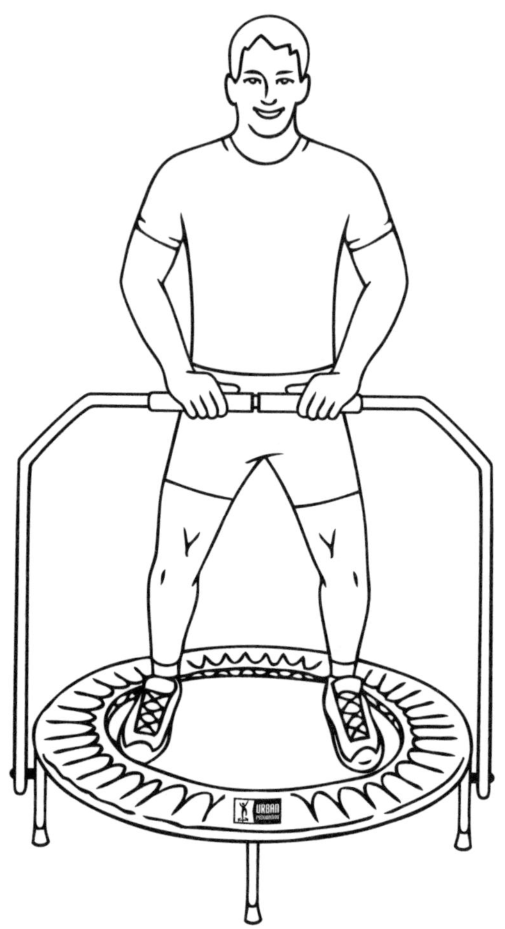

FIGURE 107. The basic stance on an Urban Rebounder.

Most exercises incorporate the horizontal plane into the exercise, such as running and swimming, and don't work against the force of gravity. They only involve acceleration and deceleration and friction from the surfaces you come into contact with. You can lift weights for pure resistance exercise, but this act can become extremely boring and can lead to injury. In fact injury of the muscles, tendons, and bones is an ongoing hazard in most extracurricular exercises and sports.

The beauty of rebounding is that it (a) takes advantage of the vertical plane, and (b) is easy on the joints, so it doesn't promote sports injuries. Using the vertical plane—with you pushing up against gravity and its force pushing upon you on the way down—makes this exercise extremely efficient. The G-force adds weight to your body (thus forcing your body to physically counter it) but doesn't pound you into the ground like running. These features have been studied by academic medical centers as well as NASA and the United States Air Force. The safety and injury-prevention characteristics of this low-impact sport have also been highlighted in their research.

One of the earlier serious investigators of rebounding was actually NASA. They were interested in using it in astronaut training. What they found is that compared to treadmill jogging, rebounding is 68% more efficient and effective. Another study done at the University of New Mexico corroborated this research. They also showed that a rebounding workout burned the same amount of calories as jogging, but that it was much easier on the joints. Studies have also shown how rebounding can help balance and coordination, a byproduct that few other exercises can offer. A study at the Hospital for Special Surgery, a world-famous orthopedic hospital in New York City, showed that participants rebounding three times a week for 20 minutes a day demonstrated a nearly 70% increase in balance and coordination. Researchers noted that this would help prevent falls that lead to contusions, hip fractures, and damage to knees, ankles, and other bones. (For more information on the many rebounding studies that have taken place, see the research section at *www.urbanrebounding.com.*)

As you can surmise, if aerobic exercise is your goal to strengthen your heart and other muscles, I could not recommend a better exercise for you than rebounding. It strengthens you systemically and even at a cellular level. It is also a wonderful core workout, meaning it strengthens the muscles of your abdomen and torso, which benefits your entire body and helps prevent spinal pain and degeneration. I don't believe in marathon workouts, though. Most people won't stick to an exercise routine if it isn't enjoyable. The great part about rebounding is that it's so efficient it doesn't have to be a marathon workout to be highly effective, and it's fun to do! As an exercise routine, I recommend three days a week for 20 minutes. (For more information on exercise routines, see the end of this chapter for resources.)

So rebounding can and should replace whatever exercise routine you have going on. However, this chapter is not really about rebounding for exercise, it's about rebounding for 60 seconds a day! Rebounding can be an outlet to the stresses of modern life that is ultimately necessary for the health of the body and spirit. It has become clear to me that rebounding on a regular basis can become an integral part of developing and cultivating a lifestyle that brings us closer to our natural homes. It is designed to serve the needs of the human body, but it also nurtures the mind.

I recommend 60 seconds of bouncing in the morning (or anytime during the day when you feel sluggish or tired) to get your lymph moving, to wake yourself up, and to get a quick dose of positive energy. After I do my 60 seconds of rebounding, I feel completely refreshed and invigorated. It also has an effect on my digestion and stools, making it easier to go to the bathroom.

The *basic stance* is the key position for the Urban Rebounding technique. All other actions come from this stance, including the *basic bounce*. If you are taking a rebounding class, it is from this position where instructor cues are given.

Focusing your eyes straight ahead, place your hands on your hips and stand with your feet slightly wider than hip distance apart (see previous illustration). Your back should be straight and leaning forward about 10 degrees, your knees should be slightly bent, and you should be standing on the balls of your feet. Your center of gravity should be kept low with concentrated intention on your body's center. The proper stance is very important to rebounding, and to having a successful workout if you are doing a full exercise routine.

For the basic bounce I recommend for your 60 seconds, the bounces are gentle and your feet do not even leave the mat. They are called basic bounces because of the internal cleansing effect such movements initiate to the lymphatic system. As I have discussed in earlier chapters, the lymphatic system moves toxins and bodily waste out of our bodies but does not include its own pump as the circulatory system does. Rather, it depends on the movement of our respiration and musculature to move it through our bodies. The basic bounce movement serves the function of acting as the body's own lymphatic pump by gently pushing the lymph through the body for removal. Simply stand in the basic stance and bounce gently on the balls of your feet such that your feet remain on the surface of the mat while you bounce.

I really cannot tell you in powerful enough words what rebounding has done for my life. I started rebounding 20 years ago when I heard about the amazing health benefits to the lymphatic, digestive, and circulatory systems. I feel that rebounding is also great at protecting from and helping reduce varicose veins (spider veins) and cellulite as well because the exercise moves lymph so effectively and efficiently. In the beginning I was jumping up and down for a minute at a time throughout the day strictly for the health benefits. I would rebound for one minute in the morning and then a few times during the day, and I would always feel a burst of energy that lasted for hours.

When I injured my knee about 13 years ago, I took rebounding to another level. I needed a workout that had all of the benefits of rigorous exercise but that was easy on my joints. In all physical exertion, I love free-form exercise where I am not locked into an activity or mechanical device, and that also engages my mind—and rebounding fit into these criteria perfectly. When I discovered that a safe, high-quality rebounder did not exist, I designed one and sold it commercially to fitness centers. I created the Urban Rebounder fitness program as well.

Today, Urban Rebounding is in thousands of gyms throughout the world and in 18 different countries and nine languages. The program has been accredited with the American College of Exercise, and the equipment has been voted in Consumer Reports' top 100 products of the year.

I highly recommend doing your 60 seconds and/or rebounding exercise routine on an Urban Rebounder. This will ensure maximum efficiency and safety. I know this, because I designed it that way.

Now go purchase an Urban Rebounder…it will change your life and the way you look at exercise.

For more information on rebounding and the Urban Rebounder, go to:
www.DOITORAGEQUICKLY.com
www.URBANREBOUNDING.com
www.JBBERNS.com

17
WONDERFUL WHEATGRASS

For 60 Seconds:
Get your daily dose of wheatgrass.

Wheatgrass refers to the young grass of the common wheat plant, *Triticum aestivum*, and is used like an herb for its nutritional and medicinal properties. It is taken freshly juiced or dried into powder, both of which provide chlorophyll, amino acids, minerals, vitamins, and enzymes, for animal and human consumption.

The consumption of wheatgrass in the Western world began in the 1930s as a result of experiments performed by agricultural chemist, Charles F. Schnabel. Schnabel used fresh cut grass in an attempt to nurse his dying hens back to health. The hens not only recovered, but they produced eggs at a higher rate than the already healthy hens. Encouraged by his results, Schnabel began drying and powdering grass for his family and neighbors to supplement their diets, and he promoted and popularized the technique from there. He marketed his discovery to feed mills, chemists, and the food industry. By 1940, cans of Schnabel's powdered grass were on sale in major drug stores throughout the United States and Canada.

Wheatgrass has not been studied nearly enough, perhaps due to the fact that a large pharmaceutical company is not going to shell out the millions needed to study naturally growing grass. Yet, the studies that exist and personal anecdotes of healing are compelling.

Some of the benefits of wheatgrass may be:

- Improved digestive system
- Diabetes prevention
- Heart disease prevention
- Colon cancer prevention
- Constipation cured
- Heavy metals detoxified from the bloodstream
- Helping menopause be more manageable
- Helping slow down the aging process
- The promotion of general well-being

Wheatgrass, like green leafy vegetables, is rich in chlorophyll. Besides giving green plants their color, the chlorophyll found in them may be a health-enhancing antioxidant. Antioxidants have been associated with the reduction of chronic disease, including reductions in high blood pressure, diabetes, Alzheimer's, heart disease, and especially cancer. Most of the health benefits related to antioxidants have to do with their role in maintaining the health of body cells and tissues.

In addition to increasing overall immunity, antioxidants interfere with some processes that create carcinogens (cancer-causing agents). Carcinogenesis is a multistep process (involving oxidative damage, DNA damage, and so on) that can be reduced or prevented by dietary antioxidants. Antioxidant activities include the regulation of gene expression in cell proliferation, cell differentiation of oncogenes and tumor suppressor genes, induction of cell-cycle arrest ("apoptosis"), stimulation of the immune system, and many others.

It is believed that antioxidants play a major role in the prevention of atherosclerosis by mopping up oxidative damage in the arteries. The theory goes that when LDL cholesterol (the "bad" kind) is oxidized, it is rendered sticky and adheres to the sides of arteries, which over time will clog them. When antioxidants are present, however, they will become oxidized instead.

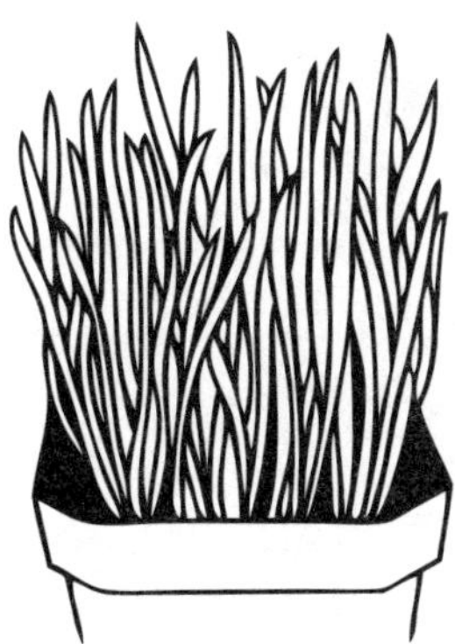

FIGURE 108. The wheatgrass plant.

Just like the sprouts of cruciferous vegetables (broccoli, cauliflower, and so on), wheatgrass benefits are best realized in young plants preparing for a growth spurt and rich with nutrients. Laboratory analyses indicate that the nutrients found in young green cereal plants vary with the stage of growth. Chlorophyll, protein, and most of the vitamins found in cereal grasses reach their peak concentrations in the period just prior to the jointing stage of the green plant. Although this period lasts for only a few days, grasses that will be consumed as food supplements must be harvested precisely during this stage of the wheat's development.

The jointing stage is that point at which the internodal tissue in the grass leaf begins to elongate and form a stem.

This stage represents the peak of the cereal plant's vegetative development; factors involved in photosynthesis and plant metabolism would be expected to increase up to this stage.

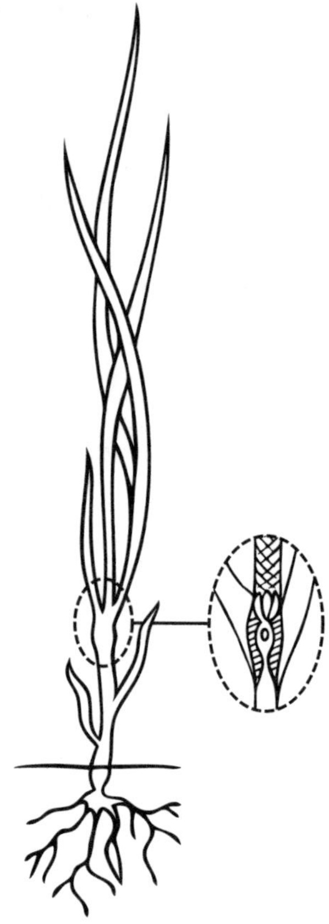

FIGURE 109. The young wheatgrass plant showing the jointing (harvesting) stage.

After the jointing stage, the stem forms branches and continues to elongate. The chlorophyll, protein, and vitamin contents of the plant decline sharply as the level of cellulose increases (cellulose is the indigestible plant fiber that provides structural stability for the growing stem).

Harvested grass is then dehydrated and made into powders and tablets. Wheatgrass can also be grown indoors in shallow trays for 10 days, which will contain similar nutritional content. Upon indoor harvest, you may put it in a juice processer and make a thick, dark green juice out of it, which is what I recommend. The nutritional content is better preserved if it has not been dried out. You can also take it as a rectal enema or implant.

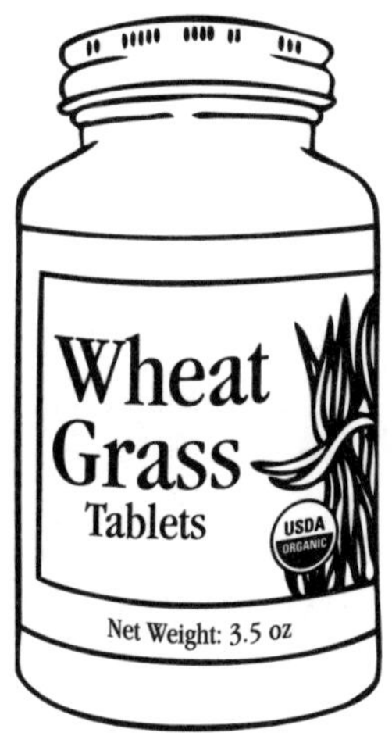

FIGURE 110. Wheatgrass tablets.

The average dosage taken by consumers of wheatgrass is 3.5 grams (powder or tablets). Some also take a fresh-squeezed 30-milliliter shot once daily. Try to consume at least two ounces of wheatgrass a day, or the comparable dose in pills, although the juice extract is by far the best because it has more live, active enzymes. (When you drink the few ounces of extract, do not swallow right away. Swish the liquid in your mouth for a minute, swallowing a small amount until all of the extract in your mouth is gone; this benefits your teeth and gums.) For more therapeutic benefits, you can take a higher dose of up to two to four ounces, one to three times per day, on an empty stomach and before meals. For detoxification, you might increase your intake to three to four times per day. It should be noted that some users experience nausea on high dosages of wheatgrass.

For more information on wheatgrass juice and tablets, health benefits, and growing your own, you may want to get the book shown below on wheatgrass. I am also making the best wheatgrass tablets available for purchase on my website, for those times when you're not near a health food store or want the convenience of taking a tablet instead of juice.

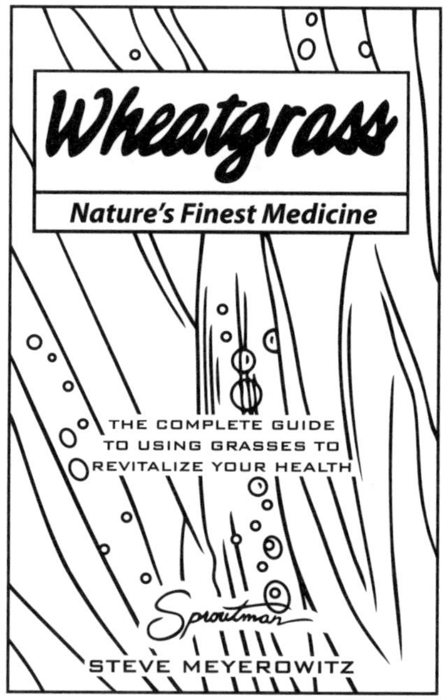

FIGURE 111. ***Wheatgrass: Nature's Finest Medicine*** **by Steve Meyerowitz.**

I really cannot say enough about wheatgrass juicing and wheatgrass tablets, and I sincerely hope that you will give it a try and see what it does for your immunity and your energy. Simply put, it will change your life (as I hope this book will!). It changed my life over 20 years ago when I began taking it, as I have a much stronger immune system, and it makes me feel fantastic. Wheatgrass is also wonderful for strengthening your gums and teeth. I get my wheatgrass juice delivered to me each day, and when I'm away and miss a few days, I really feel the difference. I have less energy, and my immune system is not as strong. There is a reason horses and cows are so strong: what do they do all day? They consume a lot of grass! Wheatgrass is a wonderful gift from Mother Nature—take advantage of it!

Take a moment to take your wheatgrass, you will thank me for it.

For more information on wheatgrass and where to purchase it, go to:
www.DOITORAGEQUICKLY.com
www.JBBERNS.com

18

THE HEALTHY WAY TO YOUR NATURAL WEIGHT

For 60 Seconds:
Carefully select your meal, eat properly, lose weight.

Eating a healthy diet can be one of the most profound ways you can benefit your overall health and the way you feel on a daily basis, as well as influence your long-term health and increase your lifespan.

People who consume a typical Western diet are often overweight and are likely to contract many weight-related illnesses throughout their lifetimes. They also are usually not receiving sufficient nutrients nor supporting adequate digestion. By consuming a proper diet, there are countless disorders and diseases you can prevent or lessen, such as heartburn/gastroesophageal reflux, diverticulitis, arthritis, diabetes, high blood pressure, stroke, heart attack, and cancer.

I believe the Taoist practice of trophology is the answer to many ills of the Western diet. Trophology is a system whereby foods are eaten separately or in very specific combinations in order to maximize digestion and minimize bacterial growth in the digestive track. Furthermore, by following its guidelines, weight-loss diets become unnecessary as appropriate foods are selected and digestion becomes highly efficient.

Throughout my 20 years of training friends, family, clients, and celebrities, I have given numerous people the trophology technique and way of eating, and they have shed a tremendous amount of extra weight throughout their entire bodies. They experienced much-increased energy levels, and their digestion, stools, and gas levels (from both upper and lower digestive tracts) improved.

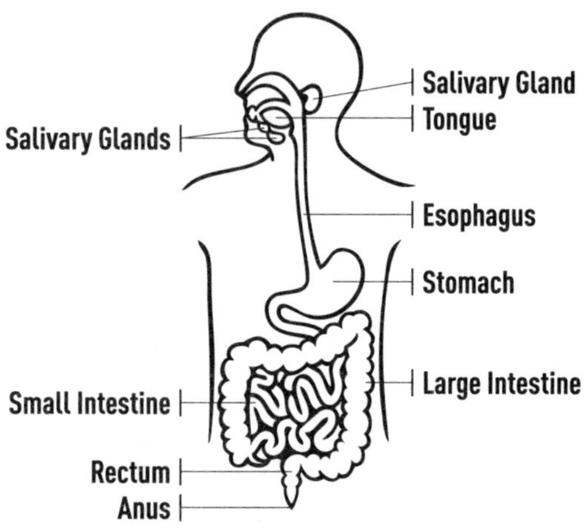

FIGURE 112. The digestive system: What we ingest must work in harmony with the mechanics of the digestive system with which we were born.

The following section lists the basic tenets of trophology, along with brief explanations. Trophology offers guidance on the following foods and food combinations:

- Protein and starch
- Protein and protein
- Starch and acid
- Protein and acid
- Protein and fat
- Protein and sugar
- Starch and sugar
- Milk
- Fruits
- Desserts

Trophology

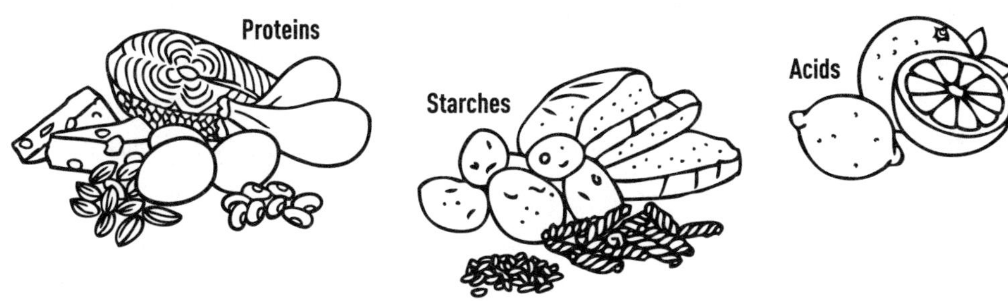

Protein and starch—Eat concentrated proteins (such as meat, fish, eggs, and cheese) separately from concentrated starches (such as bread, potatoes, and rice). A protein and starch are the worst possible combination of foods to mix together at a meal. When one eats a starchy food, the alkaline (basic) enzyme ptyalin is secreted in saliva, which begins its digestion and starts breaking down the starch. In order to digest concentrated animal protein, the stomach must secrete the acid pepsin (acidic). The problem arises when one combines a starch with a protein, because the basic enzyme and the acidic environment become neutralized, and in this environment bacteria can thrive. The undigested protein is thus left behind to produce toxic wastes and foul gases.

Protein and protein—Eat only one major type of protein at a single meal. Different proteins have different digestion requirements and can conflict with each other.

Starch and acid—Eat starches and acidic foods at separate meals. An acidic food such as lemons or oranges will stop the secretion of ptyalin; thus, a starch eaten simultaneously would not be properly digested.

Protein and acid—Avoid combining concentrated proteins and acids at the same meal. When acidic foods enter the stomach the secretion of hydrochloric acid is inhibited, which in turn inhibits pepsin secretion, which is needed for proper protein digestion.

Protein and fat—Eat concentrated proteins and fats at separate meals; if you can't avoid combining them, also eat plenty of raw vegetables to assist in digestion and passage. Fat exerts an inhibiting influence on the secretion of gastric juice. This makes fried meats particularly detrimental and will delay digestion of the meat.

Protein and sugar—Avoid consuming proteins and sugars at the same meal. All sugars inhibit the secretion of gastric juices in the stomach, so eating sugary foods along with proteins will not allow proper digestion of the protein.

Starch and sugar—Eat starches and sugars separately. As with acids, when sugar enters the mouth, ptyalin secretion is inhibited. This will prevent proper digestion of the starch. Furthermore, such a combination blocks passage of sugar through the stomach until the starch is digested. Because starch digestion is delayed, the sugar will then ferment, creating an acidic environment that further inhibits starch digestion.

Milk—Eliminate pasteurized and homogenized milk products from your diet; use certified raw milk or milk products if available (not in combination with other foods). Many studies suggest that pasteurized milk (pasteurizing removes active enzymes) is very difficult for humans to digest and is not an efficient way to get calcium. Certified raw milk is better for you, and there are many vegetables that are an excellent source of calcium as well, such as dark-green leafy vegetables (e.g., kale or spinach).

Fruits—Eat fruits alone or leave them alone. Try to eat fruits on an empty stomach. Melons are an excellent fruit as, when eaten alone, they require little digestion and pass quickly through the stomach and move into the small intestine. If other foods are combined, fruits will not pass out of the stomach until the digestion of other foods in the stomach is complete. This causes the fruits to ferment and leads to gastric distress.

Desserts—Avoid sweet starchy desserts, as well as fruits, after large meals of proteins or carbohydrates; eat sweets as a separate meal if you must. A sweet dessert combined with anything will contribute to ineffective digestion and gastric distress.

Menu—A helpful sample menu following trophology principles can be found in the book *The Tao of Health, Sex & Longevity* by Daniel P. Reid (Fireside, 1989), Chapter 1, Appendix II.

NOTE: *A food containing 15% or more protein is considered a protein; 20% or more carbohydrate is considered a carbohydrate/starch food. If only a small amount of one food is combined with another predominant food in a meal, especially if combined with plenty of raw vegetables to add active enzyme and fibrous bulk, the deleterious effects will be negligible.*

People always say to me, "JB, you consume a large amount of food, but you are always slim and look fit—how do you do it?" I then explain to them the beauty and art of food combination I learned from Daniel Reid. Trophology is a wonderful way to lose extra weight that your body does not need or want. I also feel that your digestion is greatly improved, your stools will be much better and more regulated, and your overall body will feel lighter and more supple. Please, I urge you to just try trophology food combining for 21 days. What (and how many pounds) have you got to lose?

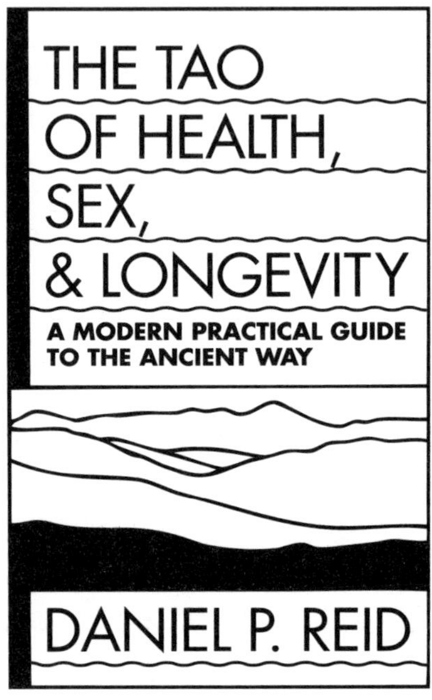

FIGURE 113. The practice of trophology is detailed in the book *The Tao of Health, Sex & Longevity* by Daniel P. Reid.

In addition to the principles of trophology, I would like to share with you diet advice I give to all of my clients. These suggestions will help you lose weight if you need to, aid digestion, and generally improve your diet and nutrient absorption.

- **When you wake up in the morning, have an 8-ounce glass of warm water with a half lemon.** Lemons are great detoxifiers, rich in vitamin C (so they boost your immune system), aid in digestion, and benefit the gastrointestinal tract. It's a great way to start the day and will make you feel wonderful!

- **No white flour or foods from sealed cans.** Try to eat fresh foods. They are much healthier for you and you will have more energy. Stay away from white flour foods such as donuts and cookies, as well as sweets like candy and ice cream. Eat natural unprocessed foods like fruits, vegetables, and unsalted nuts.

- **Before swallowing, chew your solids until they become liquid.** Digestion begins in the mouth. By chewing foods well your digestion and assimilation of nutrients should improve. As Ghandi said, "Drink your food and chew your beverages." In other words, chew until your food is liquefied, and drink liquids as slowly as solid food. This applies especially to carbohydrates, which require contact with the alkaline ptyalin enzyme in saliva to begin proper digestion. This also allows the sensation of fullness to develop so you won't overeat.

- **Try not to drink liquids during your meals.** Drinking liquids during your meals does not allow you to chew your food thoroughly and may wash down nutrients prematurely. For example, when you eat a starchy food, if you don't allow the enzyme ptyalin in your saliva to do its work, digestion will not begin properly.

- **Eat sparingly to live a long, healthy live.** Taoist principles teach that you should only eat until you are 70 to 80% full. Mother Nature punishes those who overindulge with all sorts of health maladies. The human body is not designed to handle large quantities and the complex combinations of the modern diet and the contemporary sedentary man. Furthermore, numerous studies have suggested that calorie restriction (without restricting nutrition) may elongate one's lifespan.

- **Eat like a king for breakfast, a queen for lunch, and a prince for dinner.** It is a good idea to minimize your intake at meals as the day proceeds. A classic pattern of the overweight is to do the opposite: to eat very little during the day and then binge in the evening (because they're so ravenously hungry!). In addition, having a large dinner before bed will not allow for good rest and also not allow enough time for proper digestion.

- **Avoid extreme hot and cold temperatures in foods and beverages.** This can irritate the lining of your tender digestive tract and disrupt efficient digestion.
- **Try not to consume food three hours before you go to bed.** You will get a better night's rest on an empty stomach rather than a full belly.

The wonderful part about all of the advice in this chapter is that it takes no extra time at all out of your life to enjoy the benefits of a good diet and good nutrition. You have to eat anyway, so make your choices healthy ones!

For more information on trophology and diet advice, go to:
www.DOITORAGEQUICKLY.com
www.JBBERNS.com

19
POWER OF THE MIND

For 60 Seconds:
Smile at yourself in front of a mirror.

In this chapter I would like to explore the power of the mind over the body. We tend to think of the body and the brain as completely separate entities, but the brain is an organ like any other, and it is intimately tied to the functioning of all of the systems in our bodies. It's easy to see the connection if you think about what effects mere thoughts can bring about in your body: your face flushes when you feel embarrassed; your heart races when you feel angry, nervous, or scared; your body responds when you think of something sexually arousing. But what can we do to rein in those responses and use them to our advantage?

Utilizing the power of the mind to help prevent illness is only in its infancy in terms of our research and understanding, but we are gaining knowledge all of the time. One area that has been studied more than any other is depression and its effect on human health. The psychological disorder of depression alone is linked to the following diseases:

- Diabetes
- Heart disease
- Stroke
- Cancer
- Osteoporosis
- Parkinson's disease
- Epilepsy
- Alzheimer's

We don't know for certain the pathophysiology that makes depressed people prone to all of these illnesses. Making it trickier to uncover is that there seem to be many paths that lead to the different diseases. For example, serotonin, a neurotransmitter that plays an important role in elevating mood, may keep platelets from clumping together and forming artery-forming clots. This may explain why depressed people with low levels of serotonin are more prone to heart attacks (and repeat heart attacks) than nondepressed people. Depression may also set off immune system alarms, may make the body less responsive to insulin, and likely sets off stress hormones that damage the body.

Stress in particular can take a great toll on the body. Acute stress, usually a response to imminent danger, turbocharges the system with powerful hormones that can damage the cardiovascular system. Chronic stress, caused by constant emotional pressure the victim can't control, produces hormones that can weaken the immune system and damage bones. I will touch on this in Chapter 20, The Five Rules to Conquer Fear, but will describe the effects of stress in more detail here. Basically, a stress response to something begins in the brain, and a number of neural structures are activated and exchange information with each other. Nerve impulses and signaling hormones are sent to the rest of the body to prepare for "fight or flight."

Adrenal glands are activated by this pathway and release adrenaline, which makes the heart pump faster and the lungs work harder to flood the body with oxygen. The adrenal glands also release extra cortisol and other glucocorticoids that help the body convert sugars into energy. Nerve cells release norepinephrine, which tenses the muscles and sharpens the senses to prepare for action, and digestion shuts down.

This is quite a system-wide response to deal with the presence of stress! It's not difficult to imagine how this could negatively affect your health. In addition, if this response is chronic, adrenaline and norepinephrine levels will damage the arteries over time. Glucocorticoids will remain in circulation and lead to a weakened immune system, result in loss of bone mass, and suppress the reproductive system and memory.

While there seems to be more evidence on how depressive thinking is linked to poor health than positivity leading to good health, there is also research that suggests the latter may be beneficial as well. For example, studies have shown that meditation and other relaxation techniques can counteract the fight-or-flight response that floods the body with stress hormones. Studies have shown that meditation can reduce hardening of the arteries, especially in African Americans with high blood pressure. People suffering from anxiety disorders also appreciate the lowered stress, reduced blood pressure, and slowed heart rates associated with meditation. Similarly, there is growing evidence that a meditation program can have a positive, sustained effect on chronic pain and mood, including depression and anxiety. In an even more dramatic example, initial research has suggested that meditation combined with dietary changes may slow tumor progression in prostate-cancer patients.

To meditate, a person sits comfortably and silently, centering his or her attention by focusing his or her awareness on an object or process (e.g., breathing, a sound such as a mantra, a visualization, or an exercise).

I believe that in addition to helping prevent illness, the power of the mind can help heal the body as well. There is much power in the practice of visualization. A striking example of this technique is found in the book *Zen in the Martial*

Arts by Joe Hyams. Hyams tells the story of Sam Brodsky, a kara-te instructor. Brodsky had set out to break nine 1-inch slabs of concrete with one punch of his fist for his kara-te students. When he smashed his fist onto the slabs, he broke all but two. Unfortunately, he had also broken many of the small bones in his knuckles. Doctors needed to operate, and after his hand was put back together with wires, he was told it would take 15 to 18 weeks for any kind of healing to take place. Brodsky, however, had studied martial arts in Korea and Japan and believed that the key to healing lies in the mind.

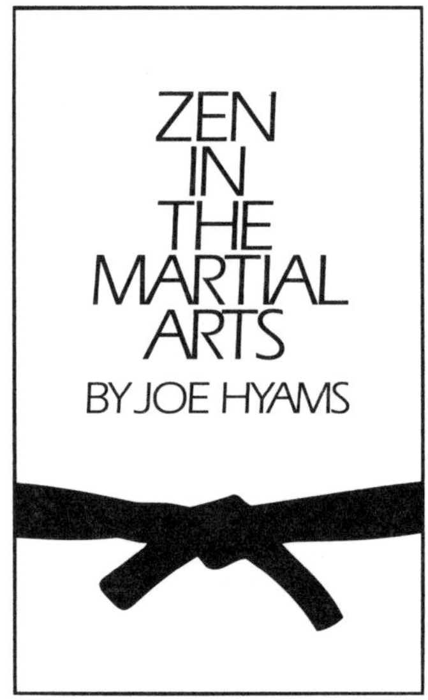

FIGURE 114. Powerful examples of using mind over matter are described in the book *Zen in the Martial Arts* by Joe Hyams.

On the night he came home from the hospital, with his hand in a cast, he began imagining that his arm was a building site with hordes of workers trying to fix it. He had quite specific imaginings of the work site, and would focus on it every night as he fell asleep. Only two weeks later Brodsky went back to the doctor, who took off the cast and said that the healing process had been quite amazing. However, now his knuckles were frozen together.

Undaunted, Brodsky went home, and before he fell asleep each night, he now visualized those same men set to work on his knuckles, sanding and lubing and repairing them until they could work. Seven weeks later when he went to see his doctor, his doctor pronounced it a miracle. The healing that would have normally taken a year took only 10 weeks!

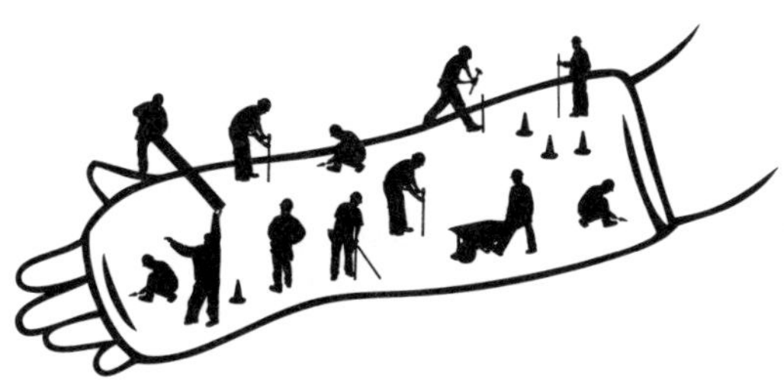

FIGURE 115. Visualize healing, and healing will come.

As a teenager I read this story about Brodsky and was impressed. Little did I know that I would need to use his technique not long afterward. During the ninth grade I was in my room doing homework. Outside my window I could hear my neighbors playing basketball, and it was too good to refuse. I threw on my sneakers and snuck out my window with untied shoelaces. When I went to dunk the basketball, I tripped on the laces and ripped ligaments in my ankle. Suddenly, I was in excruciating pain. After a trip to the emergency room, the doctor predicted it would take at least three months for my ankle to heal. However, I followed the technique just as Brodsky had, and it healed in half that time.

Another way to positively influence your life and health is by smiling! In this case you're putting the expression before the feeling, and the feeling will follow. Stand in front of a mirror—I suggest you do it when you wake up in the morning and start your day off this way—and **smile for 60 seconds.** Some studies suggest that there is a feedback mechanism in our facial expressions that influence our emotions. It can't hurt to take a glimpse of yourself looking happy as the start to every day. I believe it's contagious. I recommend heading back to the mirror whenever you feel frustrated throughout the day. It's difficult to remain angry or anxious (with those stress hormones coursing) when your smiling face is looking back at you!

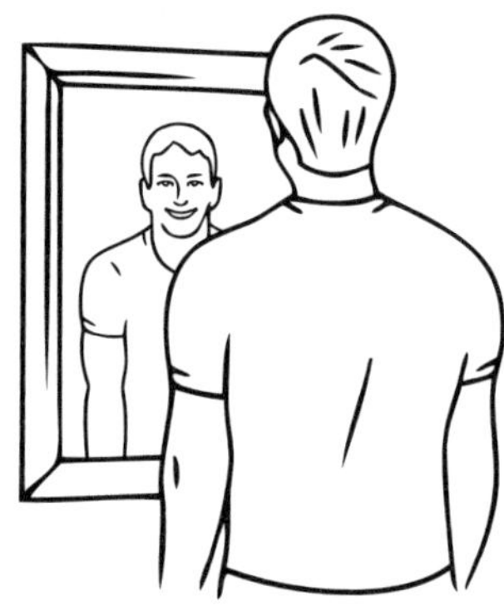

FIGURE 116. Wake up with a smile.

I realize that the technique of smiling in the mirror sounds so odd and so simple, but it should reap great rewards if you do it 21 days in a row. There is nothing wrong with talking to yourself silently or even out loud, and, better yet, there is nothing wrong with laughing at yourself and becoming ideally "light." Meaning, you will be less stressful and more enjoyable in your personality to yourself and others. You will find that in stressful situations, or on days of no stress at all, you will come to really enjoy this 60-second technique of smiling in the mirror. In fact, it is one of my best times during the day. Several times a week I burst out in pure reflexive, spontaneous laughter, where sometimes my abdominal core region even gets a bit of exercise. Try it.

Finally, I would like to talk a little about the power of focusing your mind. By blocking out all extraneous thought outside the immediate goal you wish to accomplish, you can achieve great things. Using this technique in sports is a good example. In *Zen in the Martial Arts*, Hyams tells the story of watching Bruce Lee put outstretched fingers against the chest of a man who was much bigger than himself. With lightning speed Bruce contracted his hand into a fist and punched with such force he was able to propel the man into a swimming pool 5 feet away. Bruce explained his ability by saying he was able to focus on the muscles of his body and relax everything, and then, at the moment of action, he called up *everything* to the effort.

The power of focus can take many forms. Use it to accomplish tasks you set before yourself. Personally I use it day to day, such as when I'm about to do a yoga handstand. If I focus and visualize it, I can do it; if I don't, my failure rate is much higher. Imagine what more you could do if you concentrated your thoughts and put everything into the effort at hand.

For more information on the techniques mentioned in this chapter, go to:
www.DOITORAGEQUICKLY.com
www.JBBERNS.com

20

THE FIVE RULES TO CONQUER FEAR

For 60 Seconds:
Read page 42 of *Das Energi* by Paul Williams.

"A new bacteria threatens to cause widespread illness. This is information you cannot miss! Stay with our channel to find out everything you need to know, coming up."

If you heard this, you very well might stay tuned in to your channel and wait for this clearly important and possibly lifesaving information. You would probably have to first sit through stories about current events, weather, sports, and, most importantly, countless commercials before the story would show up at the end of the broadcast. News broadcasters are highly attuned to what you're anxious about, and in their desire to get you to watch their broadcasts, they are not averse to playing that for all it's worth.

In the well-detailed book *The Culture of Fear* by University of Southern California sociology professor Barry Glassner, many contemporary problems we fear are broken down and attributed to faulty perceptions created by the media. For example, you might think that child kidnappings, teen violence, and airplane crashes are relatively common occurrences. In fact, they're not at all, but they sure make sensational headlines, so you probably see plenty of stories reported about them. Our perceptions are manipulated by the media's use of tactics such as relying on anecdotal evidence or so-called experts who aren't really experts at all on the given subjects, and showcasing isolated incidents and dubbing them "trends." Because, of course, the more scared you are the more often you will tune in to find out what you supposedly need to know to protect yourself.

In our time, I believe more than any other, we are plagued and burdened with fear. Many issues are hyped up by the media to create fear. Many fears are based on reality as well, such as the health risks we incur in our modern chemical-filled world or the transportation risks we take every day to get to wherever we need to go. We also wrestle with emotional fears, be it over our success, illness, family, or friends. We are a highly connected society in current times, at least superficially, and we must deal with constant social anxieties that previous generations were not exposed to. Our easy access to information nowadays is a great benefit, but it also creates new anxieties, exposing us to the knowledge of worst-case scenarios for whatever problem we may be dealing with. We also have fewer resources to absorb and control our fears, because society is more fractured and busier, and fewer people are finding solace and strength in religion.

The impact of all of this fear is not trivial and not just confined to our emotions. It takes a toll on our health, and ultimately on our lifespan. When faced with chronic stress and an overactivated autonomic nervous system, damaging stress hormones are released into our body on a regular basis, and we begin to see physical symptoms. The first symptoms are relatively mild, such as chronic headaches and increased susceptibility to colds. With more exposure to chronic stress, however, more serious health problems may develop. These stress-influenced conditions include, but are not limited to:

- Depression
- Diabetes
- Hair loss
- Heart disease
- Hyperthyroidism
- Obesity
- Obsessive-compulsive or anxiety disorder
- Sexual dysfunction
- Tooth and gum disease
- Ulcers
- Cancer (possibly)

So how do we deal with the fears in our lives? I believe the best antidote to fear is thinking about fear in a different way. My reading of Paul Williams' book *Das Energi* changed my relationship with fear forever. *Das Energi* is more than a book; I believe it is a life pamphlet on how to deal with fear and other controlling factors in our lives. *Das Energi* is one of my bibles for daily life. This book, particularly the passage

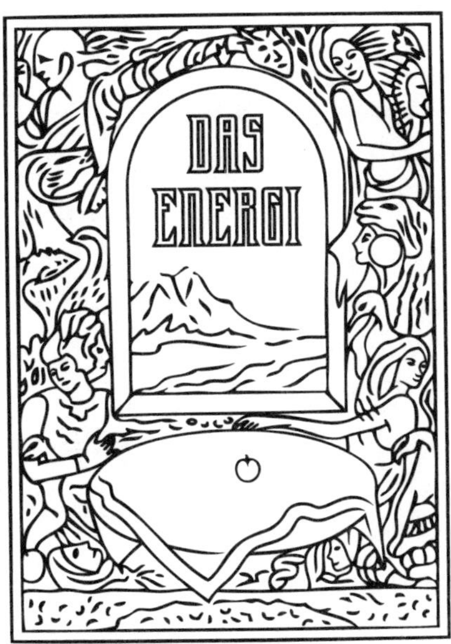

FIGURE 117. The powerful book *Das Energi* by Paul Williams.

on dealing and coping with fear, will give you confidence in your life when you clearly understand and apply it. I urge you to read the book as a whole, but page 42 (which begins, "It's hard to stop the reasoning mind,") is particularly powerful in terms of dealing with fear. Williams writes in a spare, poetic manner, and you could finish this page in about a minute.

Williams turns most people's understanding of fear on its head. Fear is not a necessary way to avoid pain or adversity; it is not necessary to be taught in this way. Rather, stoic awareness of a situation is the way to avoid or handle events you wish to keep from occurring. For example, you do not have to be *afraid* of a hot stove because you might burn yourself on it. You should simply be *aware* that the stove is hot and could burn you if you touch it.

The right approach is to think of fear as an alarm clock. When you experience it, don't dwell on it, don't let the alarm clock keep ringing: turn it off! You don't need to feel the fear anymore. Now is the time to be aware of what you need to do, to collect yourself, and take action. Accept that fear is not necessary and should be prohibited, learn to recognize it, and stop it. Stopping the sensation should become reflexive and instinctive, without deep thinking. And finally, the means to stop it is to be aware of it, respond to it, and do something about it (or accept there is nothing you can do if there is nothing you can do). Williams has reduced his viewpoint on this down to five steps:

1. **Fear must be stamped out. Accept that.**
2. **Learn to recognize fear.**
3. **Stamp it out. Reflex.**
4. **Don't think about it.**
5. **Respond. Be alert. Be aware.**

This philosophy should alleviate the dread of fear. You are not waiting for something bad to happen. You are living in the moment, free of fear. My friends, I must say that Paul Williams has changed my life for the better with his book *Das Energi*. The way he breaks down how to deal with fear is simply amazing and can be memorized—or better yet, if fully understood can become instinctive to your "basic self." The alarm clock analogy is exactly how I deal with fear in my own life, and then I follow Mr. Williams' steps.

It was an amazing teacher of mine, Professor Lanny Taylor, my speech professor, who introduced me to *Das Energi* so many years ago. Professor Taylor would read passages of the book in class, and then one day he read the fear passage, and I was "in the zone," focused and ready to apply the technique. Fear can take away so much from a richly lived life and can hold us back from achieving our true goals and dreams in life. Thank you, Paul Williams and Professor Taylor, for the alleviation of fear in my life.

For more information, go to:
www.DOITORAGEQUICKLY.com
www.JBBERNS.com

21

LIVING LIFE AS A PEACEFUL WARRIOR

For 60 Seconds:
Read this chapter.

When I was in high school, I was so inspired by the book *The Way of the Peaceful Warrior* by Dan Millman that I typed out a small card for myself to carry in my wallet. On it is a list of the most important elements of the *Peaceful Warrior* philosophy and way of life. So important is it to my day-to-day life, to the maintenance of a balanced mind and spirit, that I have kept it in my wallet for over 20 years. I lost the wallet three times, and it was returned to me three times, containing no money or credit cards but with this card in it each time. I carry it with me to this day.

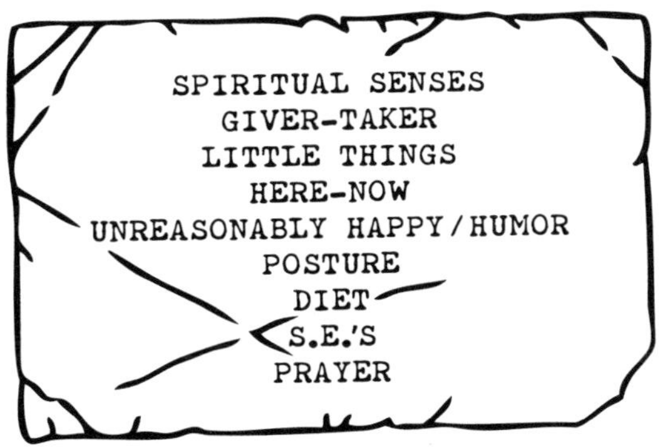
SPIRITUAL SENSES
GIVER-TAKER
LITTLE THINGS
HERE-NOW
UNREASONABLY HAPPY/HUMOR
POSTURE
DIET
S.E.'S
PRAYER

FIGURE 118. Reproduction of the dog-eared card I still carry in my wallet listing the fundamental teachings of *The Peaceful Warrior.*

While this chapter has many components, it is not meant to be followed as a daily to-do list. Rather, the *Peaceful Warrior* is a philosophy to read about and absorb, to be used as a foundation for a peaceful, happy, healthy life lived without regrets. It will take you a minute to read this chapter. Write down my list on a card and keep it in your wallet or purse. Take it out and read it every day for 21 days. Take it out when you're frustrated or upset. In time the philosophies will become internalized and a part of the way you approach life.

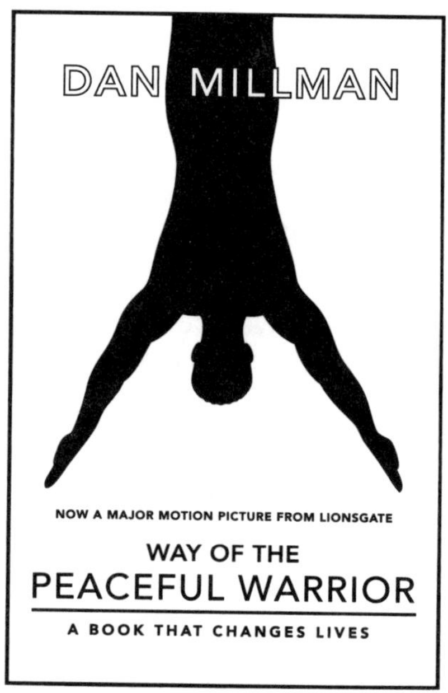

FIGURE 119. ***The Peaceful Warrior*** **by Dan Millman.**

So what does each phrase mean?

- **Spiritual Senses:** Mean what you say with all your being, speak your truth, speak from your center, speak from your senses. Don't hold back—if you feel it, declare, "I love you," or "I admire you," or "I'm upset with you." Your body and mind should act as one; your emotions and body are connected—allow yourself to feel them and act upon them.

- **Giver-Taker:** Give out what you most want to take from others and in life (e.g., love).
- **Little Things:** One of life's greatest goals should be to serve others. Try to do three little things each day to help someone. It could be a compliment, paying someone's toll, helping someone with a heavy bag, or holding an elevator door. Make sure your actions are coming from the right place, from a good spiritual sense; it should be altruistic—don't expect anything in return.
- **Here and Now:** You must live in the moment, not feeling remorse for the past nor daydreaming or worrying of the future. Imagine that someone drops a knife between your hands and you are forced to catch it; the concentration you will put on this task to be sure you catch the safe part of the knife is truly living in the moment. Pay attention to the big moments and the seemingly inconsequential ones: there are no ordinary moments.
- **Be Unreasonably Happy and Express Humor:** Even if there isn't an obvious reason to be happy, you should be! Have humor and lightness because you're alive, breathing, and on this earth for your purpose, whatever that may be. For example, if your doorbell rings and it's Publisher's Clearinghouse to offer you lottery winnings, you should be happy. However, if the doorbell rings and it's only a prank, be happy as well.
- **Posture:** Have good posture. Support your abdominals and lower back, and breathe deeply to fully oxygenate your

body and support better erect posture. Energy goes quickest in a straight line, so practicing good posture benefits both your spine and energy level. Bad posture contributes to age-related deterioration in the skeleton and other organ functioning, so particularly as we get older we must concentrate on good posture to combat these effects. Please see Chapter 1, Correct Posture: Asleep and Awake, for illustrations and posture exercises to reinforce and strengthen correct posture positions.

- **Diet:** Eat all things in moderation. Have a "see-food diet": see what you want to eat, but eat it in moderation. Your diet should be a means to benefit and sustain you, not give you cause for ill health or anxiety or contribute to aging. (See Chapter 18, The Healthy Way to Your Natural Weight, for more specific advice in this area.)

- **Spiritual Exercises:** Take time out of your day, every day, for you and only you. This will allow you to focus on your being and basic self and to regain power in your goals and who you are. It doesn't have to take long; it could be for only a minute. It could be listening to your favorite CD, meditating, practicing needlepoint, masturbating, or taking a bubble bath. The exception to this is when your body takes time out for you, meaning you get sick; during these times allow yourself to relax and heal. These are referred to as spiritual exercises because they lift your spirit and heal your mind. They help your mind and body relax and give your being more inner peace.

- **Prayer:** Be thankful and humble. You should not have to see a homeless or handicapped person or someone worse off than you to feel grateful for your life. Always remember how fortunate you are, be thankful for all that you possess, and carry that with you. You should have the Zen concept of the "beginner's mind," meaning you should have a clear and open mind and be humble and concentrate on living in the moment. This attitude does not leave room for regret or fear but builds a grateful focus and acceptance of the present time.

A further *Peaceful Warrior* concept is the idea that life is made up of three primary elements: **Change, Paradox, and Humor.** You might say that the first set of "rules" were about things you can change, while this set is for the things you cannot. If you can embrace these concepts and accept them, you will live a more peaceful, richer, less-stressed life. You must accept that life is about **change**—there is always something changing and moving; nothing stays the same. To wish that anything will stay the same is futile and can only cause disappointment and sadness. You must also accept that life is a **paradox**: it is absurd, an unfathomable mystery, and to try to figure out its meaning or rationale is a waste of your precious life on earth and takes away from the living of it. And finally, you must keep a sense of **humor** about you. There is much you cannot affect or change, and sometimes you just have to laugh about it.

Ultimately the *Peaceful Warrior* philosophy is about living your best life. This means living healthfully and allowing your body to maximize its potential. This means living in the moment and not surrounding yourself with thoughts of the past or future, with regrets or daydreams. The way of the *Peaceful Warrior* is an awakened approach to life filled with purpose and direction and allows you the motivation and fortitude to change your life and incorporate positive changes into your life on a day-to-day and moment-to-moment basis.

It was a cold day in late September, and I decided to take the New York City subway to save some time and arrive at my meeting downtown ahead of schedule. It being midday, the subway was of course very busy, and the car I was traveling on was packed with commuters. I became aware that a middle-aged man was rubbing himself against me as we all moved through the tunnel. The man was clearly and rudely invading my social space, and coupled with the foul smell coming from his clothes and mouth, it was a very uncomfortable and unpleasant situation. I was getting more and more aggravated at first, but instead of lashing out at this man or saying something in the heat of anger, I simply took a few deep (foul) breaths and took out my *Peaceful Warrior* card from my wallet. Instantly, my mind and body began to relax. I meditated on the laws of the *Peaceful Warrior* and embraced them. I gave what I wanted to take, I was unreasonably happy, I laughed, I stood straight, I relaxed my mind and body, I gave thanks, I humbled myself, I said a prayer. The time flew by, and the ride was soon over. I did not lose my cool whatsoever, and I learned in true action how to control my mind and body.

Follow the ways of the *Peaceful Warrior.* It takes just 60 seconds, if any time at all.

For more information on *The Peaceful Warrior*, go to:
www.DOITORAGEQUICKLY.com
www.JBBERNS.com

EPILOGUE

This book would not have been possible were it not for the philosophies that shaped me and these chapters. As I formally endorse all of their writings, products, and websites, I would like to provide resources here if you would like more information on several of the sages featured most prominently in this book.

Dr. Stephen Chang has clearly influenced the chapters in this book a great deal. His books, *The Complete System of Self-Healing: Internal Exercises*, *The Great Tao*, and *The Tao of Sexology* are life changing. You can learn more about Dr. Chang and Taoism on his wonderful website, *www.thegreattao.com*.

More information on Daniel P. Reid, master Tao herbalist and author of *The Tao of Health, Sex, & Longevity*, can be found at *www.danreid.org*.

Dan Millman, author of *The Way of the Peaceful Warrior*, maintains a website where he offers workshops and supplemental materials for his amazing book: *www.danmillman.com*.

Unfortunately Paul Williams, author of the book *Das Energi* featured in Chapter 20, suffered a brain injury some years ago and is no longer active (*www.paulwilliams.com*). However, I urge you to read this book in its entirety, as it may permanently change the way you look at life for the better.

INDEX

D

E

I

J

K

L